A Clinician's Guide to
PSYCHODRAMA

Third Edition

A Clinician's Guide to
PSYCHODRAMA

Third Edition

Eva Leveton, MA

Springer Publishing Company

Springer Publishing Company, Inc.
536 Broadway
New York, NY 10012-3955

Acquisitions Editor: Sheri Sussman
Production Editor: Janice G. Stangel
Cover design by Susan Hauley

01 02 03 04 05 / 5 4 3 2 1

Library of Congress Cataloging-in-Publication Data

Leveton, Eva.
    A clinician's guide to psychodrama / Eva Leveton—3rd ed.
        p., cm.
    Includes bibliographical references and index.
    ISBN 0-8261-2263-9
    1. Psychodrama.   I. Title.
        [DNLM: 1. Psychodrama.   2. Psychotherapy, Group.   WM 430.5.P8 L663p 2001]
    RC489.P7 L48 2001
    616.89'1523—dc21
                                                                    00-067913
                                                                    CIP

Printed in Canada by Tri-Graphic Printing

Contents

Prologue

When I started my first psychodrama group, I was highly skeptical. I had ample reasons. Untrained in the highly specialized techniques of Moreno's psychodrama and inclined to label such techniques as "gimmicky," I wasn't sure if I could do it, and, even if I *could*, I wasn't sure I wanted to. But the touching scenes produced by group members using dramatic techniques proved to be irresistible. I forged ahead, stumbling through many an awkward beginning, sustained by curiosity and the excitement of learning.

The time was the early 1960s; the place, San Francisco—a place only beginning to feel the stirrings of those active iconoclasts who were to revolutionize therapy. Family therapists were being trained at the Mental Research Institute in Palo Alto; Eric Berne's seminars attracted crowds of young people; we flocked to see a man named Fritz Perls demonstrate Gestalt techniques; we listened with a combination of timidity and excitement to such phrases as *dance therapy, art therapy, body awareness*—words wafting our way from the steamy hotsprings of Esalen, California. It was a time of experimentation, a time when many were learning and few qualified as experts.

When one of the larger day-treatment centers in San Francisco wanted to start a psychodrama group, it was difficult to find anyone to run it. A friend suggested that I try. She had known me long enough to know that, in addition to being a psychologist at U. C. Medical Center, I had been active in the theater—acting, directing, teaching. She also knew that I was interested in learning more about group therapy. I was interested—very interested—but scared. It occurred to me to read everything I could, fly to New York to Moreno's

Institute, take a crash course; but I knew that I would not really profit from such extreme measures. I don't learn fast. And I have to start with what I know and can do in order even to begin to formulate the problems and questions with which I can use help. I decided to try it if it could be labeled an experiment. I wouldn't charge for the first six months, while I worked out techniques based on my acting experience. The staff agreed.

I remember sitting on the stage of a large gymnasium facing about thirty people, most of whom looked forbiddingly tense, anxious, and withdrawn. Usually, sitting on the stage with my legs dangling into the pit got me over my stagefright. I used to teach drama that way, leaping up to demonstrate if necessary. Not this time. I talked a little about the experimental nature of what we were doing. That helped. From now on at least I didn't have to be a "psychodramatist." And then I taught a beginning acting class. Simple sense-memory exercises right out of Stanislavsky. One client showed us in pantomime how she cleaned her room; another, how she prepared a meal. I saw that the act of performing these tasks was satisfying. Clients were rewarded by therapists who also felt intimidated by the notion of performance. I asked them to do pantomimes of arriving home after attending the center. Climbing the stairs, fumbling with the key, throwing down the coat, grabbing a drink, sitting down, a blank expression. Time after time either there was no one else living there or the meeting was embarrassed, self-conscious. After everyone had participated, we talked about how we felt. The empty, lonely feeling became a shared experience. There were tears. Faces looked softer. I knew I would be continuing with psychodrama.

Following the work on stage, the center's staff led sessions that gave me a chance to learn something about group therapy and to evaluate the results of my techniques. Of course, I began to read voraciously—Moreno, first and last. (I really think he and his wife Zerka have said everything there is to say in those phenomenal volumes (*Psychodrama, Vol. 1, 2,* and *3*, Beacon, N.Y.: Beacon House, 1946; revised 1964)) and their many other publications. I also read pamphlets, chapters, anthologies, anything I could get. I attended workshops given by the Morenos as well as by Moreno-trained individuals, including Dr. Richard Korn. At the same time, I was caught up in the surge of active techniques involving encounter, art, and movement.

I have remained eclectic. My own timidity rose to gigantic proportions whenever I expected myself to be a "something"—a psychodramatist, a facilitator of encounters, a movement or art therapist. I rebel against labels. I still rebel against the unquestioning use of another's vocabulary. I didn't want to pretend or promise something I couldn't deliver. I could promise that we would be using techniques from the theater to work on problems involving the psyche; therefore, *psychodrama* still seemed the most appropriate name. I couldn't promise a "classical" Moreno-style but I knew I couldn't proceed without crediting the man who originated this powerful work.

This book is an account of my experiments. For the last decade, I continued to lead at least two weekly psychodrama groups in day centers or hospital wards, to give workshops and teach classes in the use of psychodramatic techniques, and to develop their use as an adjunct to clinical practice with individuals, families, and groups. My goal is to let you know as much as possible about my experience in using the techniques: my hesitations, my questions, my conflicts. I would like this book to help give you the flavor of my process in leading psychodrama groups in order to increase your own choices.

As I wrote this, I found myself more and more cramped by the voice of my conscience: *You can't do this, Eva. If you're going to call it psychodrama, you have to do it just as the Morenos teach it. You can't use just some of their knowledge, like taking what you like from a smorgasbord. And you can't just describe what you do. You have to theorize. You have to examine the theoretical background of Moreno's work. Compare it to Freud's. Feed in Lewinian field theory. Lead them through group therapy and clinch it with a fusion of Greek catharsis and the encounter group experience. They won't accept you, Eva. They won't respect you.* If I could find a way to ignore these lectures I'd feel more at ease. Of course, I can't. I'm timid about writing this book. Afraid of all the criticism. But I want to take the risk. My hope is that I can leave the theorizing to others for the time being. My wild dream is that Moreno will say, "It's alright, Eva. I'm delighted that you could use so many of my concepts, and that you acknowledge my work in developing them. Feel free to use only those techniques that fit your style and don't worry about the rest." Hopes and dreams don't always turn out—that's the risk.

Most of the techniques described in this book were originated by Moreno and a few were begun by me. My goal is to provide the

Most of the techniques described in this book were originated by Moreno and a few were begun by me. My goal is to provide the reader with an informal compendium of psychodramatic techniques and to describe in some detail my style in applying them.

EVA LEVETON
February 1977

Sometimes things turn out better than expected. After the book was published, Zerka Moreno wrote to me, and we began a spirited correspondence which resulted in some of the changes in the present, revised edition. I felt privileged to make her acquaintance, even more so when she later included my book, with a special dedication to J. L. Moreno, in his collected papers at Harvard. All in all, a delightful process to gain a degree of legitimacy!

Since 1977, I have continued to use psychodramatic techniques in groups and families, as well as with individual clients. Milton Erikson's use of hypnosis, story, and metaphor greatly influenced my clinical practice. I was surprised by the similarities between hypnosis and psychodrama, a subject to be discussed further in this book. I also spent time in the Southwest learning about American Indian rituals. Both trance work and ritual reinforced my conviction regarding the foundation of psychodrama: the human need for an arena where feelings and fantasies can be enacted in an atmosphere of group support.

As of this writing, a new development has occurred in the field: drama therapy, a field that began much the way I did, dedicated to unifying theater techniques with psychological growth. Some of the new warm-ups, as well as some clinical examples, are drawn from my work teaching psychodrama to students in the Drama Therapy Department of the California Institute of Integral Studies in San Francisco.

EVA LEVETON
January 1991

volume, translated into many languages, has also made its way around the world. I am honored to be included in the continuing development of the Morenos' work.

My own development has continued as I became a core member of the Drama Therapy Program at the California Institute of Integral Studies, where I taught—among other courses—psychodrama and the case seminar for the past fourteen years.

As my own techniques ripened, I am more and more concerned with following as a most important aspect of directing. I will be discussing this emptying process, readying the director for receiving the protagonist's cues. Zerka Moreno's recent emphasis on surplus reality—and what are theater and psychodrama except that— interests me. When I was young, the theater was a refuge. Now I trust the power of surplus reality to provide comfort and guidance for those who use these techniques. Recently, the *double* has been explored by several psychodramatists interested in giving the protagonist an ally, someone to slow down the action if necessary, and suggest ways the protagonist might proceed more safely. The present revision will discuss these developments and add some thoughts about the similarities and differences between psychodrama and drama therapy.

EVA LEVETON
March, 2001

A note about pronouns: times have changed since this volume was first published and the general use of the masculine pronoun is no longer acceptable. Since I feel that the use of such terms as s/he interrupt the flow, I have chosen to alternate the use of masculine and feminine pronouns as I saw fit, hoping—but not always succeeding—to achieve a fair balance.

1

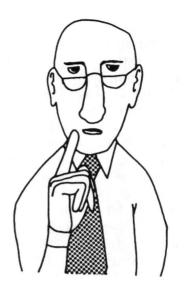

Who's in Charge?

There is a strong division among therapeutic orientations. Who's in charge? Does the hour belong to the therapist or to the client(s)? If the responsibility is shared, how do they divide it? The far left is tired of talk therapies that leave the therapist in a fairly passive role, listening to his client. Instead, they look for activities which will teach lessons through experience rather than thought. The director often emerges as a strong figure in charge of coordinating the group's activities. The far right—their loyalty to Freud unshaken and confirmed by training institutes and analyses—maintains that insight alone produces change in the human psyche and that the only true methods for achieving it involve a strong one-to-one client-therapist relationship that results from the transference of the client's emotions from past and present circumstances to the analyst himself. Here the directorship—and there are Freudian psychodramatists—is subtle, nondirective in character. In the middle are the many solution-oriented therapies from behavior modification to symptom-oriented workshops which often neglect the imagination in favor of skill training. Most therapists, however, cannot be classified as radicals or conservatives. They are eclectics, who choose to compromise between these extremes, choosing the theories and techniques which best fit their unique style of doing therapy. In the present chapter, I will discuss the strategies of directing that have formed the base of my own eclectic practice.

Playground director, psychodrama director, theater director—all operate with the same paradox. *Be spontaneous. Lead a play session. Direct the creative effort of the actor. Take charge of a group and teach its members to be spontaneous and unafraid to role-play important conflicts. Encourage spontaneity, but if someone tries to take over, let him know that he can't, lest the others be resentful. Encourage spontaneity, but if too many are spontaneously reticent, do something about it. Encourage spontaneity, but keep the group within some bounds and limits.*

Although it has made great gains in popularity in recent years, psychodrama is often new to a given setting. Even in settings where psychodrama has been used before, it is often regarded with hesitancy and fear on the part of the regular staff. One of the director's first obligations may be to arrange training where, in an informal and enjoyable structure, the staff can be warmed up to the new technique. Staff training and demonstrations can minimize problems as well as help create the therapeutic alliance that will continue to be a vital support as the group develops.

The director of a psychodrama must be able to model the spontaneity she wishes to elicit and to find ways of showing the group what can be done. She is facing people whose expectations vary greatly. Some think they have come to watch a spectacle. Others are afraid of being humiliated by a public display of their weaknesses. Many are interested in this potentially entertaining new form of learning something about themselves; very few have even the *least* idea of how to participate. Continuing with the paradox, the director must find structures which will enable the group members to spontaneously express feelings by role playing. The process of deciding what structures to use requires sensitivity to both individual and group behavior.

Moreno refers to the group "tele," the underlying dynamics of attraction and repulsion among the members. Human groups, like other animals, tend to find leaders, scapegoats, and preferential groupings based on these dynamics and groups vary greatly in their tele. The selection of mates and friends presents continuing problems of inclusion and exclusion. Tele is the term Moreno uses to describe the group members' relationships to each other—their commonality, their differences, their attractions and repulsions, their closeness and distance. He is not talking primarily about the content of these relationships—several are younger siblings, several have alcoholic mothers—although this will emerge. Rather, he is talking about the invisible string that binds some members although they may never have laid eyes on each other before, and the invisible rays that seem to keep others from even beginning an encounter. Tele is what makes some groups work smoothly and others stumble along. Tele is what operates when someone chooses a group member he has never seen before to play his father, only to find out that this person resembles his real father both in the way that he relates to him, and in some of the details of his own personal history. The director's sensitivity is important here. When she works with the members of the group she must be sensitive to their preferences. The selection of the role of a stern father will have one kind of consequence if, in the group, the "father" and son are close, and quite another if they are distant, which is why the protagonist's own choice is usually the best guide. Whenever possible, psychodrama can help group members to become more flexible in their relationships, to become aware of their tele, to renegotiate, to show aspects which change their place in the pecking order. What follows are some methods I use to assess the tele of any new group.

When my psychodrama groups are part of the program of an ongoing institution—psychiatric ward, probation department, school—I usually make it a point to talk to someone in touch with the members of my group before I meet them. I begin by gathering background information to help me choose the warm-up and prepare me for possible further work. My "contact" may be able to tell me much that will help me in choosing the type of warm-up to use and the type of work the group is ready for. I try to find out something about the group atmosphere—whether it's depressed and gloomy, rebellious, efficient, hardworking, or eager. I am always interested in any problem of concern to the group as a whole: a staff-client conflict; the departure of an important member; conflicts about house or institute rules. My informant often provides me with valuable information about individual group members—who has been the center of attention or the butt of the others' resentment, who seems interested and ready to work, who is just sitting and observing. Armed with such information, I am already a few steps away from arbitrary decisions.

I make it a practice to spend a few minutes before the group begins, talking with group members, making warm, informal contact while assessing the group atmosphere: which members seem shy, which members seem to be interested and eager to know me, what relationships exist in the group. Who will work today? Who will double? Who will play the various roles required in a given scene? What will we work on? When I compare my behavior in a regular group-therapy structure to my behavior in a psychodrama group, I find myself taking a great deal more responsibility for the group's activities in the latter. Throughout the group, I am looking for those members of the group who seem eager to work, emotionally in touch with something that is going on. They are the emotional leaders, the ones who will help me by tuning in to the mood of the group, making suggestions for scenes, volunteering as protagonists.

Information about the group also helps me develop realistic expectations of our work. A slow, quiet group can be termed successful if most of its members participate even with only a slight show of feeling. A more lively group can be expected to role-play more actively. The more realistic I can be in my expectations, the freer I will be to "hang loose," to encourage and validate the group's productions, rather than pull and tug in a direction which the group members can't or won't reach. All of this information describes the group tele.

My warm-up will depend on what I have learned thus far. If the group is reputed to be shy, somewhat depressed, and resistant to working, I may start with the simplest of warm-ups (asking each member to think of a question he could ask someone else in the group; asking each member to say a sentence he has enjoyed hearing from another member of this family, for example). My goal is to build confidence by giving everyone a chance to participate successfully. Building on this warm-up, I carefully avoid asking anyone to work, unless he is ready. Because any rejections I collect will add to the listlessness of an already depressed group, I may continue the warm-up for several more rounds. The group members' responses, verbal as well as non-verbal, will give me my first rough map of the group's tele. Who responds to whom, positively and negatively. Who is sitting next to someone that they contact as they react to what's going on. Who is alone. Who shakes her head disapprovingly. Eventually, someone will show me that he wants to work further and I will be able to proceed with the central enactment.

The greatest task facing the strong director is that of remaining sensitive to the group so that she is not a dictator. My decisions are based on information the group gives me, my informant's discussion and my own perceptions. If the group's reaction makes me question this information, I ask for further response from group members before proceeding. I may have suggested the wrong warm-up due to my particular lack of tele for a given group. If the group's responses are halting, listless, boring, I may then double for a group member, saying "What is this she's asking us to do? I don't want to do it. It's like nursery school. It's boring." If I get agreement, I will change the warm-up. The group members will be able to guide me to a more appropriate theme.

As director I must be aware of my own feelings as well as those of the group. When I sense discomfort in myself, I must do a quick check to see if it's something I've brought to the group—something personal and only marginally related, or if my feeling arose from the group's process. I may want to tell the group what I'm feeling and ask if anyone else feels the same way. When I sense discomfort in the group, it is important to check it out with group members. This constant checking of the group's reactions as well as my own provides the most reliable safeguard I know against insensitivity and arbitrary rule. I find it helpful to have eye contact with as many of the group members as I can during any one session. I pay attention to any movement or noise in the group as clues about a member's emotional involvement in a given scene. (They may, of course, only provide information about the hardness of the chairs—but it's worth checking.) The non-verbal messages I exchange with the audience during a given scene add to the group's cohesiveness. A group member sees that his director cares about his reaction, that not only those in the enactment have the director's attention.

The success of any psychodrama depends on the selection of the protagonist. In my own experience, the most auspicious scenario presents me with a small group—twelve to fifteen high-functioning individuals joined in a common activity related to their own growth—whose warm-up has revealed common themes. Because I am well in touch with the group's tele, I observe the group member's stronger responses both to the theme and to each other during the warm-up. At the end of the warm-up, one or two group members volunteer to be the protagonist and, as they tell us what they want to work on, it becomes clear to all of us that one of them is our protagonist. I have only to confirm the group's selection. There is no guarantee that such a smooth transition will occur. In large groups, there may be five or six volunteers for the protagonist role. In small low-functioning groups, finding a protagonist may be like pulling teeth.

Moreno popularized the use of sociometry for the selection of the protagonist. In short, this means that the group members vote for the candidate they want. Most often this is done by the director's lining up the candidates after they have stated what they want to work on, and asking group members to stand behind the one they want, or perhaps to touch the protagonist or someone who is touching the one they would choose. In a small group, the group members may simply talk about which person might be most appropriate. I have been reluctant to use sociometry because for me, and for some others in each group, the process risks memories of popularity contests—like the nightmare of being last to be selected for a team just after I came to the United States at the age of eleven. Only after watching other directors who do not share my personal difficulties and could present the group with the choice confidently and cheerfully, was I able to use this process, and for a large, high-functioning group, I recommend it. Once the group members have selected a protagonist, they will have a stronger stake in supporting his work than if they are simply following the director's lead. In a small, low-functioning group, however, sociometric choice may be difficult to achieve. The fear of rejection and conflict will make members reluctant to choose. Here, the director, using her best indications of tele and the themes that arose during the warm-up, will encourage a protagonist and invite the group's support.

Once the protagonist has been selected, the director must make an important transition in her own role. Up to now she has been the one responsible for the group's movement. From now on, the protagonist is. I have made this statement so strong as to be somewhat misleading, because, of course, the director is still in charge of the group. The difference lies in the way she experiences the work. From the moment the protagonist has been selected, she must empty herself as much as she can, so that she can be receptive to the protagonist's story, his mood, his verbal and non-verbal cues. At best, the experience is one where the protagonist and the director become so seamlessly related that the process is effortless. The director, instead of directing the protagonist is following him. At every juncture, she senses his needs and helps him enact a part of his story and select others to help him and then show them how to proceed. This shift—from directing and remaining in charge of the group to following and remaining empty and open to the protagonists's needs may be the key to the development of a psychodrama group that helps produce growth and change in the protagonist, the auxiliaries, and the audience.

During the enactment phase of psychodrama, one of the director's most important jobs is to oversee the selection of auxiliaries, or helpers, to the protagonist's scene. Her sensitivity to the group tele will help her make decisions that range from letting the protagonist choose his own cast—which always works best in a high-functioning, flexible group—to assigning staff members or other group members to play particular roles. In a group of high-functioning individuals, tele will enable the protagonist to choose someone whose character style resembles that of the person he wants portrayed. In a group of individuals who have less ability to function flexibly, such as a group of adolescents, or severely disturbed people, it may be important to include staff who can function as auxiliaries to help the protagonist capture his particular drama. Staff members can play the dreaded parents and teachers in an adolescent group, for example. Staff members can play a cheerful, brusque role in a group where depression reigns supreme. The director's decisions about auxiliaries, as well as the cues she later provides for their playing a particular scene are crucial in determining the success of psychodramatic work. Obviously, a protagonist who asks that his mother be rejecting will not be able to work on his problem if she is played as nurturing and supportive.

With a group whose members have shown an interest in working on their problems, and who receive me with some vitality and curiosity, I can pay more attention to the protagonist without risking that other group members will feel excluded. I can tailor my warm-up to the spirit and tele of the group without concern about their ability to participate. My choice for a warm-up is often dramatic (to portray, in a few sentences, the most difficult character in your life; to portray an authority figure such as a staff member, teacher, or doctor evaluating you). I may interrupt the warm-up in order to begin to work with an individual and then continue with the warm-up's task. In this kind of a group I don't have to worry so much about feelings of rejection, and depression. I can work with one individual for a short period, and, watching the tele of the group, continue with the warm-up, and work with another.

The director can be instrumental in keeping up the group's energy. A buoyant, enthusiastic group may lose energy during a verbal warm-up or during a painful scene. There is little an individual group member can do to bring group energy back up. The director can help by commenting on what happened, go back to revitalizing physical activities (as demonstrated in the non-verbal warm-ups), or change the scene. The director's awareness of the group's energy level is vital. There is no reason that the group energy has to remain high and buoyant at all times. Many very productive scenes have an effect of quieting the group, making members thoughtful and reflective, or sad. But when group members start yawning and voluntary participation begins to decline, the director must know how to revive the group.

I have experimented with the role of director trying—at times—a more non-directive approach, in the hope that directorship would emerge from the group itself. I might then be freed to sit back and contribute as I saw fit by playing a role or doubling. Such experiments convinced me that a psychodrama group is vastly more productive with strong directorship than left to its own devices. The directorless group—or the group that uses a director only as a consultant—spends a great deal of time overcoming initial resistances, negotiating what is to be done and how to do it. In a training group getting together for a set time period to learn about group dynamics and psychodrama, this kind of slow motion look at resistances may be a productive part of learning. In most of my work, however, I prefer to use my energy to provide strong directorship for structuring psychodramatic work to sitting back as the group struggles with its resistances.

The strong director helps encourage spontaneity by providing the security of an authority figure. The role is like that of the parent or teacher of young children who allows group members to feel: *I can play, I can try whatever silly thing I want to because there's the director keeping an eye on us; the director won't let the others hurt me and she'll stop me from hurting others; I can try whatever I think is right, the director will tell me if it isn't.*

The strong director helps members express feelings and personal conflicts by structuring the work. The group member feels: I *have something I want to talk about but I don't know what I want to do with it, I don't know if I should ask the others to play roles in my family, I don't want to ask someone to double for me. Perhaps I can bring up my problem and the director will figure out a way to work on it.*

The strong director gives permission for a great many things that group members would like to do but because of shyness and reticence, don't. The director helps the group member pick the others who are to participate in his scene. She may ask the protagonist to portray his feelings as dramatically as possible, to yell if he wants to, to put his tender feelings into words, to prolong a scene—in each instance giving permission, validating the group member in a difficult task.

As the most important person in the psychodrama group, the director makes all the major decisions concerning the activities and participants. She shapes the work by deciding how the room can be used most effectively and modulating the intensity of the scenes. She can assign many of her tasks to others in the group, but she is the one ultimately responsible. Because she has such a powerful position, the director is extremely important to the protagonist who often begins with a feeling of shyness and embarrassment. The director's physical presence reassures the protagonist well after he is committed to the scene. One protagonist, for example, whose psychodrama portrayed the early loss of her mother, pleaded with the director, who had walked across the room, "You're not going to abandon me, too, are you?" Afterward, she said that she had been half joking but felt immensely relieved when the director came back to her side.

One might suppose that the director's powerful position would lead the protagonist to become dependent on her, to seek her out for further attention either in or out of psychodramatic sessions. However, that is rarely the case. Because psychodrama is a complete event in itself when it is done correctly, the protagonist does not leave with unfinished business. While other therapies make the therapist a

participant in the client's life, the psychodrama director merely
arranges an event that allows the protagonist to look at an aspect
of his own life more intensely without playing a major role himself.
A psychodrama has a beginning, a middle, and an end. When it is
over, the protagonist is left to mull over what has happened as he
goes on with his life. Perhaps if the director were to have a series
of individual sessions with the protagonist, it would be different. But
in a group, the protagonist can be expected to leave the director
behind with the rest of the psychodrama.

When the director senses that the work is not finished, she can
help the protagonist arrange for follow-up. I have found it useful
to have most of the relevant staff of a psychiatric hospital attend my
sessions because they will have a sense of what is left over with a
particular client. In a college setting, students usually debrief each
other. Whenever the director feels closure is hard to achieve, she
can direct the group discussion to explore ways to be of further
assistance to any members who are in pain. The fact that she leaves
the responsibility for further care for the protagonist to others usually
frees the psychodrama director from the strong transference relationship formed by other therapies.

During an enactment, I may make non-verbal comments on audience members' sadness, anxiety or tension, usually by quickly mirror-
ing the physical position or facial expression. After the scene, I often
check these impressions out. For example, I may say, "John, you
seemed really tense during the last scene. Did you feel tense? Did
the scene have some relevance for you?"

When I began to lead groups, I felt great pressure to "get the
show on the road." The longer I've worked, the more I found that
a slower rhythm is vastly more productive. In her most recent book,
Zerka Moreno talks about developing a kind of zen buddhist attitude
toward her work. Perhaps it is the wisdom of the older woman
clinician—referring to zen as the key to working with students. For
me, too, the non-attachment of the buddhist is the closest description
of the feeling of inner emptiness and peace that is the key to successful, and often slow-paced work. It's true, there is no blare of trumpets
followed by a dimming of the houselights in preparation for a drama
which unfolds before the undividedly attentive audience. What happens usually starts with a quiet conversation which grows in intensity
and may even unfold into an intense drama. But the drama can be

interrupted to clarify misunderstandings or to change the focus to an audience member who has burst into tears. We move according to the rhythm of the work.

How much control does the director have? The question reminds me of one of the oldest jokes: "What animal in the jungle does the lion eat? Anyone he wants." The director does have a great deal of power. We have already learned that every major decision in a psychodrama is made by the director. Since the primary goal of the psychodrama is to create a situation in which the protagonist can behave spontaneously without help from her automatic, well-defended social persona, it follows that psychodramatic techniques increase the protagonist's vulnerability. It is very important, therefore, that the director be aware of the immense responsibility she carries. Psychodrama has many of the characteristics of an altered state (see "Trance and Psychodrama," Chapter 14). Just as individuals in altered states require others, usually not in an altered state, to guide them, protagonists need to rely on the director for psychological safety.

What, then, are the dangerous waters in which the protagonist may find herself? And what can the director do to help the protagonist with his fear of loss of control, humiliation and embarrassment, of being unable to integrate the psychodrama with his everyday life? Uncontrollable crying or anger can be stimulated by a given scene. In a college setting, for example, a student began to portray his suicidal ideation so realistically that the director walked her to the student health service after the group. On a psychiatric ward, a client in one of my groups regressed visibly during an argument with a partner who apparently reminded her of her father: in the middle of a dating scene, she suddenly rolled back her eyes and told us she was five years old taking a shower with her dad. I was able to bring her back by gently touching her and asking her to look at me, and, after a moment or so, to tell me who I was. After she was able to do that, I asked her to look around the room and make eye contact with those group members she recognized. Slowly she did so and became reoriented. By slowly reconnecting her with the present, we brought her back, but it had been a close call.

The director can also make mistakes that have lasting consequences. One man, for example, was encouraged by the director to kick the wheelchair of his chronically ill mother. Paying attention

to the enormous burden the mother's illness placed on the protagonist's childhood, the director had ignored his unresolved grief. The
guilt feelings that arose during this session were not resolved for
several years. In another group, a psychotic client was doing a scene
in which another woman, who played his social worker, was so funny
that he smiled for the first time in the months he'd been at the
hospital. The director felt encouraged. It looked like a transition
had been made. Three or four months later, however, the director
was surprised to see the same client looking morose at a Christmas
party. After some hemming and hawing, the client asked, "How can
you tell if a person is out of control?" and reminded the director
of the scene where he had lost control and smiled, humiliating
himself completely in front of the others. He had, of course, gone
back to his previous, uncommunicative, style. The first director led
his protagonist to what he believed to be a healthy reaction, rather
than following him to a more authentic response. The second failed
to check the protagonist's reaction following the enactment. In both
cases, the director was more concentrated on her own feelings than
those of the protagonist.

Feelings of anger, tenderness, grief, and sexual desire can be
aroused during a psychodrama. In a day center for psychotic clients,
I became worried when a client showed us her murderous rage
toward her landlord. (In those days therapists were not yet required
to involve the police in such a process.) I was able to make arrangements for follow-up, which insured that she did not go home unac-
companied until those feelings had abated. In another group, a
husband became so angry at his wife that he threatened to go home
and break the furniture. At a day center, an older man became
romantically attached to a young woman who had played his daughter in a scene. The resulting complications required the staff's attention for the following months. None of these events can be judged
as entirely negative. Important feelings were brought to the surface
for each of the group members. But each situation needed special
care because it contained an element of danger. The beauty of
psychodrama lies in its effectiveness in laying bare deep feelings.
The risk lies there as well.

These war stories are told to demonstrate the powerful forces
inherent in psychodrama. There are more subtle difficulties as well.
An abused client may not be able to integrate a scene in which

she is yelled at. A client with sexual difficulties may find himself overstimulated by a scene that takes place in the bedroom. Although she will find nine out of ten sessions smooth sailing, the director must be aware of the power of psychodrama to retraumatize the protagonist.

The director can demonstrate her ability to help the protagonist maintain control during the warm-up with comments such as, "We can start the scene here, and if you don't like how it's going, we can stop at any time," or "If the scene is not going in a way that works for you, you can always let me know what bothers you and we can change it." It is important to realize, however, that though such comments suggest the possibility of flexibility and control, the protagonist, caught in the midst of her own life drama, seldom uses such measures. There, reactions that might later disturb her seem normal. That is the difficulty.

The director's sensitivity, however, will help her set up scenes that are congruent enough with the character of her protagonist, scenes which, though they stimulate spontaneous behavior and new solutions, do not go too far afield. If she is intent on following rather than leading, her awareness will help her detect the scene that is taxing the protagonist. Sensing danger, she can arrange for auxiliaries who introduce more control (in a bedroom scene, someone rings the doorbell; when two siblings are fighting, a parent walks in). She can go back to the past where the protagonist had better control ("You told me you and your brother used to get along OK. Let's see a scene from an earlier time, so we can see what you guys were like then").

There are times when the psychodrama director permits others to direct a scene. The protagonist herself, for example, may wish to explore her material by directing others in a scene about her life, and choose another member of the group to play herself, a maneuver which allows her some distance before taking the risk of entering the drama as herself. Some groups abound with individuals eager to lead psychodramas, either because they are students eager to learn, or individuals prone to taking responsibility, or persons inclined to challenge ongoing directorship. I encourage other directors to participate in my groups. While they are directing, I have a chance to observe the group or perhaps to play a part in a scene. My first priority, however, is the overall directorship of the group. Even when others are directing, I am in charge. It is up to me to provide a bridge between scenes by different directors. It is up to me to help the group understand the separate scenes. In the event of negative consequences, it will be up to me to deal with them.

In addition to her clinical responsibilities, the director is responsible for the aesthetic quality of the session. Psychodrama directors who come from the theater are more likely to have developed an awareness of aesthetics than directors who come from the clinical field. Most clinicians, if challenged, would probably respond that the aesthetics of a psychodrama are directly related to the type of person or problem used in the scene. If what they express is aesthetically pleasing, fine; if not, so be it. However, though the personality of the protagonist determines a major portion of the aesthetics of the scene, the director still must shape it into an aesthetic whole.

What is meant by aesthetics in psychodrama? Can there ever be an element of artistic wholeness in a theater that is improvised for reasons utterly unrelated to art? My answer would be that aesthetics do play a role. Aesthetics have to do with transforming the chaos of spontaneous response into a harmonious whole. When the director uses her eyes and ears to achieve a sense of balance in a production whose participants are unaware of its wholeness, she is controlling the aesthetic element. A psychodrama that fails to achieve a sense of wholeness—a sense of beginning, middle, and end, when scenes or emotions are cut off, or change willy-nilly—leaves both audience and participants with a feeling of dissatisfaction. The psychodrama has not transcended everyday life; it has simply duplicated it. Her aesthetic sense helps the director transcend the material presented by the participants, shape it into a scene which, like a play or a movie, has some universal meaning.

The director makes many creative decisions. By determining the length of each scene and modulating the intensity of the work, the director is helping to write the play with the protagonist as the leading character. In exploring themes important to groups in sociodrama and in shaping each individual scene, the director becomes an author. Directors use behavioral validation or negative feedback by moving about the stage area, encouraging one kind of behavior, softening another. Her decisions about how many people to include in a scene and how long each character can remain on stage must take aesthetics into account. If the work doesn't hang together, if it is disjointed, the director will lose one of the most important parts of her cast: the audience.

The director's aesthetics often go hand in hand with her clinical skills. When she discourages repetition, explores deeper versions of the truth, encourages imaginative play, she is often helping to shape scenes that will be remembered like a play or a movie. Of course, when aesthetic and clinical skills are in conflict, there is no question that the clinical side must win. Otherwise, the psychodrama would be arranged primarily to please the director or the audience rather than to help the protagonist. But the director can often prune and shape the work as it develops before her eyes, and both clinical and aesthetic motives will be served.

Teaching students to become directors is not easy because directing is essentially different from other forms of participation in a psychodrama. Students often believe that they can familiarize themselves with the territory by participating in psychodrama as doubles or role-players and by being members of the audience, but that is not enough: directing has little in common with helping or watching. The most important difference lies in the responsibility of the director. An audience member has no responsibility except to attend. A role-player must take responsibility only for playing his role in a way that is helpful to the protagonist with the help of the director. But the director is responsible for the whole process. She often helps choose the protagonist and helps him to isolate the scenes of his drama and helps him find group members to enact them. Her judgment moderates the intensity of the scene, and, afterward structures feedback that will help achieve closure.

At the same time, the director must have a feeling for what is going on in the audience, because the audience will give her valuable cues (if the audience is distracted, things are not going well) and because she may want to select additional helpers from the audience, such as doubles or new members of a scene. Further, because most groups are time-limited, the director must keep an eye on the time. In my experience, sessions often proceed most successfully if the warm-up takes up no more than a fourth of the allotted time, the protagonist's enactment about half of the time (here the director must be careful to use the time to help the protagonist wind down from any intense feelings engendered by the work before he stops), and the last quarter of the session is left open for de-roling and feedback from the role-players and members of the audience to help everyone achieve a feeling of completion.

The reader will understand that leading one's first psychodrama is the psychological equivalent of soloing in an airplane—the novice must watch an almost overwhelming amount of material and keep the plane aloft at the same time. I have found it helpful to teach directing in stages. It makes sense in a class, for example, to let students develop and lead warm-ups. Many students can use past experience in acting classes and theater games as well as their own creativity to choose a warm-up appropriate for the group. As he leads the warm-up, the student begins to develop a sense of time. Later, if he is ready, he can begin to make the transition to selecting the protagonist. The third and final step is directing. Most students become a little worried and inhibited at this point, certain they can't call up the appropriate techniques. At that point the teacher can act as coach, asking the role-players to freeze while she calls the director-student over to the side and consults with him. After checking whether he'd like to continue, the teacher can codirect with the student. Of course, the teacher must walk softly to avoid upstaging her student with her more experienced and authoritative manner. In a short time, a cooperative relationship develops between the two directors—a little like two parents raising a child, I suppose—and help the student experience something of what it's like to lead a psychodrama before he solos.

A PSYCHODRAMA CLASS: SOME EXAMPLES

The following examples illustrate the use of psychodrama as surplus reality. A wonderful bit of creative imagination occurred when a student set up a scene at the lake she used to visit as a child, a time when nature had been her most trustworthy companion. She set up her house in some detail—bedrooms, kitchen, dining room—and then selected one person to play the lake, located outside of one of the bedroom windows, and another, a rather well-rounded pregnant woman, to play the sun that was rising on the opposite side of the stage area. Throughout the psychodrama, the lake beckoned and glowed and the sun radiated her warmth. At the close, there was a poignant moment when the protagonist told both lake and sun how much they sustained her. When talking with anyone about times when they felt alone in the world, it is easy to get caught in their experience of scarcity. This psychodrama illustrated vividly that non-human companionship, too, can keep the soul alive.

Greg, a young man, lost his father to a brain tumor when he was thirteen years old. Now, he is married and the father of an infant. During a warm-up, asking the group to develop a fantasy situation using their families of origin, he got in touch with his sense of incompleteness because he had lost so many members of his family before he was grown, and he developed a fantasy of introducing his child to his family of origin, living and dead. He arranged a meal with wine and cheese around a wooden table in a house in a small village in Italy. His mother sat between his deceased father and her second husband, his father's brother, a successful physician and political radical. As his grandmother gave his non-Jewish wife the once-over, his grandfather had a chance to tell the same old stories about "when I was a boy and watched the shiksahs on the other side of town." Tensions arose between Greg and his stepdad, whose advice he prided himself in ignoring. Greg spoke to his sister, another radical, about his wish for more closeness and his feeling that he was judged for being less political. Everyone gushed over his winsome baby. In a moment of tenderness, he thanked his mother for keeping the family history alive with her photograph albums, collections of letters, and festive occasions, and gave her some pictures of his wife and child to add to the collection. Most of the people in the fantasy were already dead. This scene had brought them to life again, with a poignant, generous spirit. Afterwards, several members of the class expressed a wish to belong to a family like Greg's.

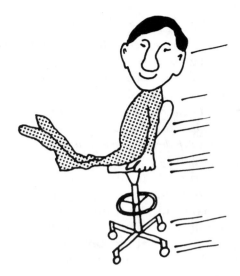

2

Seating Arrangements

Moreno describes a mouth-wateringly appealing setup for psycho-drama: a gently sloping semicircular seating arrangement for the audience, a series of wide platforms to bridge the space between audience and a stage which is equipped with light and sound effects that facilitate the recreation of a great variety of settings. Needless to say, I have yet to run into either a hospital or therapy center—not to mention clubs or schools—where even an approximation of such a setting exists. The usual accommodations vary. There may be a middle-sized room with rows of chairs and a desk, a classroom; a room with chairs arranged in a circle, a group therapy room; a room with desks and chairs arranged in a "U" or "banquet" shape, a conference room; or a vast auditorium with a small, badly lit wooden stage and rows of ancient chairs arranged in front of it. The latter may have been used as a gymnasium at one time. Usually its half-empty wooden floors make for a thunderous theatrical entrance for any late-comer.

The ideal setting rarely appears in reality and, though desirable, is not necessary. The basis of psychodrama is improvisation or make-believe. Any space can be turned into a living room, a courtroom, or a garden. Any space can become a stage. I often react negatively to the rooms provided for my groups. It's partly because I'm a rebellious, cantankerous individual overly sensitive to structures and rules. *Oh, a conference room—this is a place where you're supposed to talk, brainstorm, to SIT. No way to see anyone's body. The regularity of the circle in the group therapy room spells uniformity. No room for chaos. No expectation that there might be "a scene."*

I learned to transform my dissatisfaction into a search for something new. I started by asking people to rearrange the room in a way that would be comfortable, leaving some room for a stage area. I soon learned that this was an excellent warm-up activity. In fact, I was communicating something relevant. The message goes something like this: *I'm your leader and if I feel irritated by the way this room looks, I admit it. We don't have to accept things the way they are. In this group we can change things. There's room for some chaos here. It's not a free-for-all, I'm still in charge, and I'm mainly asking you to seat yourself where and as you want to. This is a place where we can play around, have some fun, make some noise.* Most rooms carry a message: "Be smart." "Be sensitive." "Relax." "Watch the show." The message will often add to the group inhibitions unless it is labeled or counteracted in some way.

By now you will have guessed my first requirement for seating arrangements: flexibility. A bare room with pillows or light and easily movable chairs is preferable. Most of the time, people in my groups sit in a circle using the middle as the stage area. I encourage informality. I move around a good deal myself and am glad to see others do so. If some people want to sit on the floor, I usually join them. I discourage "hiding" (sitting directly behind someone else, watching from the doorway). However, if I discover that any closer commitment is difficult for a particular group member, I prefer coming and "hiding" to not coming at all.

My own movement in the group usually proceeds as follows. I start by sitting somewhere in the circle and tell the group something about myself. Whether the group is new to me or not, I know that they're watching me keenly and I believe that some information will help them make more sense out of my behavior. Then I start the warm-up. From here on in, I try to remain flexible. I want to be able to sit next to any individual who seems to be working on something that could be developed a little further. In the following example, the warm-up was to express irritation with a member of the family of origin.

Emily says, "I'm talking to my mom: 'Mom, stop treating me like a baby. I'm twenty-one-years-old. It really makes me mad when you do that.' " I get up from my chair and sit next to Emily, asking the person next to her to change seats with me. "I'm your mother, Emily, and I can't help worrying about you. You just don't take any responsibility," I say.

Emily proceeds to argue with me (now playing the role of her mother) for a bit. When she says, "We do this over and over again and it's always the same," I drop out of my role and ask her if she is willing to come back to this problem and work on it after the warm-up. When we do, group members are already familiar with the basic conflict, and roleplaying and doubling is facilitated. When a scene is set up in the middle of the room, or in any "stage area," the protagonist (in this case, Emily) is often reluctant to step into the limelight. I try to help bridge this transition by moving into the center with Emily. I ask her to describe the living room where she talks with her Mom. As she sets the stage, I usually sit or kneel next to her so that the other group members aren't blocked from seeing. When she begins to talk with her mother, I move back to the periphery again and usually remain standing somewhere in the circle so that I can move around, asking others to participate in the scene or participating myself when I want to.

It is very important to me that the stage itself be a flexible area. Even in rooms equipped with a regular stage, I may want to move to a circular or semicircular arrangement of the group either on stage or in the auditorium. The room itself may provide various areas, each appropriate for a particular scene setting. During a single psychodrama session, a different area may be used to suit each different scene. A family drama can be set in the part of the room where a sofa and some upholstered chairs are located; a later scene may make use of the large space in the middle as the social room of the hospital with group members moving on and off stage as they spontaneously take roles in the scene; the last scene of the day may take place in yet a different area of the room where a desk is suitable for use in a job interview.

Working with distressed patients in psychiatric wards often means working with individuals who have talked very little for weeks, who move rigidly and slowly, who seldom look at the others in the room. To ask one of them to step up on the stage, speak loudly enough to be heard, and show us what bothers her is asking her for more than she can give. Her dramatic statement is her withdrawal. At the same time, she may want to come out of her quietness and tell us something about herself if we don't make it too hard. I may start my work with her by sitting next to her and talking quietly. If I get any sense that she wants to work, I may ask other group members to come and sit near her, and take roles in her scene. This strategy often helps the reticent, but it may lead to frustration for other group members who are sitting too far away for easy hearing. If this is so, I encourage the group members to move closer to the stage area. I explain to the group that it's hard for Mary to talk much louder at this time, and that it would be more expedient for the other group members to come closer in order to facilitate better hearing. The physical closeness of the group members often acts as further emotional support for the protagonist.

Groups are not always filled with reticent patients. On the contrary, psychodrama groups are often attended by individuals whose energy and sense of excitement increases with the thought of being on stage. Adolescents filled with the drama of their conflicts with unsympathetic authority figures often fit this category. People with a love of acting or some actual acting experience may already associate the stage with an opportunity to show emotion, to get in touch with fantasies, to try on new roles. If a stage is available, I will use it to work with these individuals; they often infect others with their enthusiasm. Afterwards, I may shift back to "the round" to work with less stagestruck group members.

Flexibility is all. If group members can sit where they like, move when they need to, spontaneity is increased. If the stage can be anywhere, the imagination is challenged and stage fright, often a reaction to the focus of attention of an actual stage, diminishes.

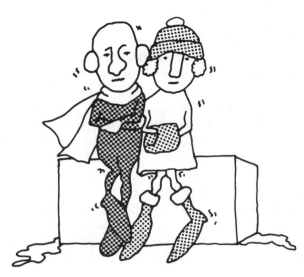

3

The Warm-Up

As a family therapist accustomed to the intense focus of a family in crisis, the idea of a warm-up was difficult for me to accept when I started. Who needed a warm-up? Pain is strong and each one of us lives out a multitude of psychodramas. I could see no need to use our precious time in a potentially artificial group activity. I thought: *the thing to do is to plunge in. Go in with the expectation that group members want to work on their problems, ask for volunteers, and find a dramatic form which will help produce insight, catharsis, and then try various alternative solutions.*

By now, the reader will have guessed that therapeutic optimism of this sort is bound to run up against resistance. Each risk of self-discovery is bound by paradox. *I want to change but I don't want to risk anything new. I want to risk something new but I'm afraid I might change. Anything's better than what's happening now. Anything's better than the unknown.* A psychodrama group stimulates additional resistances particular to acting, role playing, psychodrama, and staging. *Do I have to be able to act? I'm not an actor. I can't be phony, pretend to be someone else. Do you have to perform? In front of an audience? They'll just make a fool of me, make me act out my problems and then ridicule me. Who is that new lady? A client? Oh, she leads it. What's she going to make us do? I heard they really got emotional here last week—Anne left crying that day. I don't want that to happen to me. Not in front of the whole group. I'm just going to sit quietly and hope she doesn't look at me.*

I learned that groups are different from families in crisis who come in to the session with a common concern. Whether they are familiar with each other or are strangers, group members enter the session from a wide variety of different places. Each time it meets, the group needs to experience something that forms them into a whole. I soon realized that both the group members and I needed a warm-up, a relatively neutral activity that would allow us to learn something about each other. By relatively neutral I mean a warm-up that gives the participant a choice about the amount of personal disclosure she is willing to make.

The warm-up should also illustrate the dramatic nature of the group work as opposed to other—possibly more familiar—talk therapies. In my psychodrama groups, I discourage talking about an event whenever I can, preferring—right from the beginning—that participants show us by doing. Rather than talking about her father, I encourage the client to portray him; rather than describing a crisis that took place at home, I ask her to pick some members of the group who could play the important roles.

The following are examples of verbal and nonverbal group warm-ups. These exercises will provide the director with valuable information about the group tele. It will show her which members are willing to participate, give her clues about whether there are any problem areas common to several members of the group (always a preferable choice for later work), inform her about group members who react strongly to each other. By setting up a warm, easy going atmosphere, the warm-up also gives the director an opportunity to dispel misconceptions about psychodrama—such as the demand for performance—by encouraging shyer members and rewarding all responses. The best warm-up relates to other activities that bind the group together. In groups with a common goal, these are easily thought up.

A group of teachers, for example, can be asked to think of a specific teacher-pupil conflict. I may begin by asking the group to form pairs. The next task is a simple one. Each member of a pair has to choose to be either No. 1 or No. 2. When everyone has made a choice I ask the ones to be teachers, the twos to be pupils, and request that each pair decide on a specific conflict. Each pair is given a short period of time to work it out. The director may want to walk around, taking a look at the different pairs and then, perhaps, ask one to demonstrate, depending on the confidence level of the group. Whether or not the conflict is seen by the other group members, the content of the work can be developed further later on.

Many of the warm-ups in this section suggest that individuals or pairs demonstrate their work in front of the whole group. The warm-up can also be structured to begin in a small group that is only observed by the director who will then find a way to use the material for further work.

On a psychiatric ward, a community meeting with compulsory attendance precedes my weekly session. Often, the nurse's description of what went on in the meeting will provide a warm-up. The content of one meeting, for example, concerned planning the day-clients' activities on weekends. A lot of apparent helplessness and loneliness had appeared to be beneath the surface, but the clients' discussion had avoided painful emotions by centering on plans for weekend picnics, bus rides to the park, etc. The warm-up consisted of asking each client to imagine coming home from the hospital that Friday night and showing us what happens, using chairs and existing doors for scenery, while speaking out loud whatever thoughts and feelings came to mind. The warm-up gained dimension and poignancy, as one experience affected the next, and the feelings of isolation and helplessness no longer remained below the surface.

The director who lets herself imagine a warm-up can choose from so many possible contents: the time of the year, a particular holiday, a common bond of the group, family relationships, the newspaper. Any content can be used to start a sentence, to give to a small group for preparation of a short scene, for creating a sculpture.

There are times when little or no information about the group's background or recent experience is available. No warm-up suggests itself, and as I look around the circle of expectant faces, I feel less and less sure of what I want to do. And here, of course, it is important to remember that the director, too, needs a warm-up. For a reason that may occur to me later or that I may never know—I lack tele, the automatic bridge to the group's needs, with this particular group. I must find one of the ways that's always served me—and they will differ with each director's personality—to relax, to open myself to what's going on with the others, to lead me out of discouragement and into discovering the needs of the group. For me, this means I need to breathe deeply, to relax my body, and then, perhaps, to tell the group that I'm feeling at a loss and I need help. On another day, I may find that after relaxing and giving myself a chance to start over, I can make a humorous remark that will lead me to a better connection with one or several group members. Once I have improved my own state of mind, I will be able to develop a more appropriate warm-up. At such times, I choose techniques gleaned from encounter groups, acting classes, party games, body movement work—in short, from wherever I can find them. Some examples follow.

VERBAL WARM-UPS

The first warm-up encourages verbal participation, and stimulates body movement. The body is often neglected by psychotherapy where only words connect therapist and participant(s) like the ballooned conversation in comic strips. When group members handle a ball—imagined or real—and move to pass, catch, or throw it, the group becomes enlivened and human contact enlarged.

Ball-Toss

Directions: "I have a ball. While it's in my hands I can talk. Without it I can't. Whoever catches the ball—whoever has it in his hands—has to talk. The others can't." The next step involves an important decision for the director. What will she say before she tosses the ball to someone else? Solutions range from "Who are you? Tell me something about yourself," to more structured tasks such as "I'm your mother, what have you got to say to me?" or "If you were an animal (an actor, a character in a fairy tale or television show, a plant, etc.), what would you be?" After I have asked my question, I toss the ball to the person whose response I want, telling him to throw it to someone else when he has answered me. If two people get into a prolonged discussion, throwing the ball back and forth, I may try to catch the ball in order to ask that each person try to include someone new when he asks his question or makes his challenge, so that the warm-up reaches as many members of the group as possible.

Discussion: This is an excellent warm-up for a large group in a large room such as a gym or auditorium, in which the ball can be rolled or tossed freely but it can also be used in a very small room—as long as the ball remains imaginary, in which case the therapist mimes the ball.

Questions

Directions: "Look around the room in silence for a few minutes. Find someone whom you don't know very well and ask that person a question."

Discussion: This is an unthreatening warm-up, easily performed by a timid group. In leading this warm-up, it is important to accept all questions and answers even though they may appear undramatic and superficial at first. Once the ice is broken the director can move to deeper issues. I may make the transition, saying, "That's good. Now I'd like you to try a slightly different type of question. From now on, I'd like you to ask questions relating to feelings." If the group members are new to each other, I may add, "As you looked at the person you chose, you probably had some idea of how she felt. Maybe you could tell her what you thought and check it out with her." If strong feelings are present, I may say "You have strong feelings about the person you want to question. Maybe you could describe them to her and find out how she responds." As individuals address the warm-up, the director has a chance to ask questions of her own pertaining to feelings a group member may have about another's life, his family members, friends, or job. Once these questions are answered, it is easy to plan work for the rest of the group's time.

Feedback

Directions: "Think of a sentence you'd really like to hear (wouldn't want to hear) from someone else in this room, or from a friend or member of your family. Be that person and say the sentence."

Discussion: I often use this warm-up on the psychiatric ward with clients who have been too depressed to participate in other activities. With very little effort, clients often find themselves opening up to intense emotional experiences. One woman, for example, responded by saying, "I'm my own son, and he's saying, 'I still care for you even if I don't write.' " The scene that followed allowed her to express her withheld feelings about him.

This warm-up also gives people a chance to air complaints. When the remarks we all dread hearing are aired, laughter often ties the group together: "I'm my wife: 'You're late again, Jim.' " . . . "I'm my son: 'Dad, why can't I have the car tonight?' " . . . "I'm my mother: 'I've waited up for you all night.' " . . . "I'm my boss: 'You're fired.' " The blueprint for later enactments are clearly laid out.

Talk to the Place Where You Are

Directions: "Pretend that this social club (school, office, psychiatric ward, therapy center) is a person standing in the middle of the room. Talk to him. Complain, demand, plead, etc. Maybe you want to thank him for something."

Discussion: A director new to the group can learn a lot about a group's common experience from this warm-up. In a group where I already have information about ongoing conflicts, this warm-up can provide a forum for airing them. For example, a social club may be having difficulty getting members to do the work necessary to support its functioning, an office may have endured recent clashes between its liberal and conservative elements, a psychiatric ward may have sent a group member to another hospital, etc. When such conflicts are in the air, this warm-up provides a platform for airing them and using them for further work.

Introductions

Directions: "Be someone in your family (someone important to you) describing you in a sentence or two." This task has many variations, e.g.: "Choose another person in this group. Be that person talking about you"; "Be your therapist (teacher, group director, boss) and tell us about the progress you are making."

This warm-up must be demonstrated immediately after the directions are given, as it is difficult to describe and words may elicit confusion easily avoided by an example. Rather than answering questions, I usually say something like, "Let me show you what I mean. I'm my mom. Let me tell you about Eva. She is a whirlwind! I never knew where she's going to turn up next! I wish she'd settle down. We count on her, though. She's there when we need her."

Discussion: This warm-up acquaints the group with role reversal, provides a great deal of information as well as easy, natural transitions to further scenes. Verbal, extroverted group members often enjoy portraying someone important in their lives, especially if they know in advance that the portrayal does not have to be long and detailed.

An interesting variation is to ask the group members to introduce themselves, telling us two truths and one lie about themselves. Permission to tell tall stories often results in hilarious play and the curiosity aroused by the puzzling direction may last for a long time.

Childhood Play

Directions: "Think of your favorite game or pastime when you were a child. Imagine yourself playing the game, what you looked like, sounded like, what your surroundings were—until you can really see and feel yourself as you were then." A three to five minute silence follows. "Now, staying at the age level you've just thought about, tell us your name—you may have a nickname. Remember, we don't know how old you are, and what your favorite game is."

Discussion: This warm-up facilitates the awakening of vivid childhood memories. The participants must be encouraged to make their contributions in the role of the child that experiences the game, rather than the adult recalling it. Other childhood experiences useful for further work will naturally arise. This particular warm-up facilitates work in the area of early socialization—the joy of being accepted, having a friend, the dreaded rejections by other children, by the coach, the teacher, the scout leader.

The following warm-up also recalls vivid childhood memories.

Time Travel

Directions: "Imagine yourself as a child. Choose whatever age first vividly suggests itself to you. Give yourself some little time to really place yourself at that age, so that you can re-experience what it was like to be you then. You may close your eyes if you wish." A three to five minute silence follows. "Now, I'd like you to stay at the age you've just been imagining and tell us as that child how a typical day passes for you. Start by telling us when and where exactly you wake up and go on from there."

Discussion: All warm-ups involving childhood memories stimulate recall so vivid that the participant, who hadn't realized how exactly he had stored his early experiences, is surprised. This phenomenon has consequences for the director. Participants may need more support and encouragement because, without their usual adult defenses, they may feel particularly vulnerable. Most of the time the memories produced are recalled with a mixture of feelings—some anxiety, some remembered warmth—and the participants share a delightful and real sense of rediscovery.

There are also times when an individual recalls an important childhood experience so vividly that she may appear to become stuck there and need the director's help to make a bridge back to her present adult role. The director can ask the individual to make some then-and-now statements. ("Then I felt little, now I don't feel little but I still feel insecure; then I was never mad, now I get irritated easily.") Other methods are (1) a second exercise that duplicates the warm-up except that this time she is to use the silent time to think herself back to her present self and environment; (2) to see if she can form a mental image of herself as a child and then another of herself as a grown woman and to describe what she sees; (3) to ask her to recall her present self and then to have a conversation with the child-self using an empty chair. (See "The Empty Chair," chapter 14).

A variation of this warm-up is to travel to the future. "Imagine yourself at this same time next year . . . in ten years . . . 20 years . . . and tell us something about yourself."

Another childhood recall technique I use quite frequently, "Writing with the unaccustomed hand," is described in the nonverbal warm-ups section of this chapter.

Then and Now

Directions: "I'm going to give you a sentence and I want you to fill in the blanks. The sentence is, 'In this group I'm a . . . (I feel . . . , I want . . . , I can . . .); outside of this group I'm a . . . (I feel . . . , I want . . . , I can . . .). It doesn't matter how you fill in the blanks. I'll start by saying, 'In this group I'm a psychodrama director; outside I'm a gardener having a hard time with the deer who eat my beans.' "

Discussion: This is another technique which helps break the ice in a shy group. Its disadvantage is that it is not dramatic and a transition is necessary before role playing can begin. Exploring material brought to light during the warm-up will help to dramatize it.

Next Step

Directions: "I'm going to give you a sentence to finish. The sentence is 'The next step I want to take in my life is. . . .' "

Discussion: I have used this warm-up successfully when I have learned someone in the group has just taken a new step in his life. I may, for example, hear that Henrietta, who has just graduated from high school, has applied for her first job. With her permission, I will discuss it in a little more detail with Henrietta in front of the group, and then proceed with the warm-up.

Also on the "talky" undramatic side, this exercise provides a safe beginning. The director might follow up by asking each group member to tell the group what would be involved in taking his own next step, what would favor his doing so, what would hinder him, and use the answers to set up further scenes.

Another Path

Directions: "Today I want you to try something really different. I want you to fantasize a dream existence. If you weren't who you are, who would you like to be? Where would you live, what would you do with yourself? You can choose any life-style you've ever heard about."

Discussion: In a group where spontaneity and willingness to deal with fantasy exist, this warm-up can be quite exciting. The Walter

Mitty in each of us takes pleasure in being given an airing. Group members often develop a sense of spontaneous play in this warm-up which can be extended by scenes in which the individual chooses others in the group to help her role-play her fantasy existence. In one of our groups, for example, a famous ship captain conducted interviews with other group members applying for jobs on his ship for its impending world cruise; in another a millionaire chose to assign roles to two women who portrayed famous movie stars fighting over his attention.

Treasure Trunk

Directions: The director can start this activity with a story about treasure chests or trunks to provide the context for the warm-up. It is quiet, conducive to reflection. To set the scene, I like to describe two treasure chests, one in our attic, and one downstairs on our glassed-in porch. The one on the porch is very, very old. It's made from dark oak that would be splitting apart if it weren't for the iron bands that have held it together all these years. The iron work that decorates the chest tells us that it once belonged to two people, M.C. and A.H., who were about to get married in 1791. It comes from Westphalia, Germany, where my father's family lived for at least one hundred years. I've filled it with important things. It used to hold the leftovers from my parents' household: an old silver-service, some vases, picture frames, old photographs, bits of lace, a jar filled with buttons, my father's cigar box, my mother's combs and brushes. It also held documents. After these items had become absorbed into my own household, it became our Christmas box, holding the playdough ornaments the family has made since the children were small, decorations made in school, favorite ornaments and cards. This treasure chest contains family sentiment past and present together with items whose use and/or origin is lost in the mysterious past.

The treasure chest in our attic is different. It's only about seventy years old, a trunk covered in tattered linen with metal fittings, lined with chintz with a removable tray lined in the same faded print. For years now, it has been our theater trunk. It holds clothes, wigs, masks and makeup from my old theater days, from the children's school performances and Halloween and other costume parties. There's a white beard and wig I'm particularly fond of, made of white string and a lot of fat cardboard commas, and a vest made from an old fur coat that's served as a medieval forester's costume as well as part of a gorilla. This is a treasure chest of the imagination.

Directions (after introduction): "Each of us has a collection. It could be in a cigar box, an envelope, a corner of a closet or a desk. All of them are full of treasures, some meaningful and others that puzzle us when we take them out. Why save this? Why not get rid of it?

"Here's what I want you to do. Go over one of your collections and take something out of it. Something you just don't need anymore. And throw it away. We have quite a collection of throwaways here—a huge jar of buttons attached to a clotheshorse in perpetual overdrive, obscene earrings left by an uncle, a collection of old bills, notes for a Ph.D. thesis, a rag doll. Just come over here, take it out of the trunk and dispose of it in whatever way that appeals to you. (Here the director pantomimes the action.) When you're done, someone else will follow. We won't talk until after we've finished. Go ahead."

Discussion: During the discussion, the director asks each group member to describe the item he got rid of. With a high functioning group, the members can be asked to talk as the object and describe themselves. This exercise can be followed by another exercise in which group members approach the chest to take something out that they want to keep.

Colors

Directions: "Think of a time in your life that you remember clearly and intensely. It can be any kind of event or time, happy or sad. Assign a color to that time. Then find a partner to be in that scene with you. Tell your partner something about the event and tell her what the color you have chosen means to you."

Discussion: Color often adds something intense and intuitive to the scene. Example: Marni remembers attempting to climb a glacier in the Swiss alps. The color is silver. It reflects the intense cold of the mountains and also something about the quality of her fear. Her partner has to encourage, help, and scold her into continuing.

Life Is Easy . . . Life Is Hard

Directions: "Imagine a line down the middle of the room that represents a continuum. At one end, 'Life is easy.' At the other end, 'Life is hard.' Walk around, up and down, trying out different parts of the continuum and talking with some of the others you find there until you find the right spot for you."

Discussion: Having found his spot, each participant tells how he got there. A popular way of mapping any continuum relevant to the group, this warm-up can be used to map the members' degree of desire to be in the group, in the setting, their feeling of illness or health, etc. It permits emotional release from joy to intense complaining. Further development can pit individuals or groups from each side against each other or use members of the same side to double for one another.

Family Fantasy

Directions: "Imagine your family at any time that you recall vividly. Give yourself some time. Imagine how old you were, what you looked like, what the others looked like, what was going on, where you all were, etc. (Allow a few minutes to elapse.) Now, let's see if you can make a switch. Put that same family picture of yours into a fantasy scene, a scene, in other words that could take place anywhere, anytime."

Discussion: This warm-up gives permission to play out in surplus reality fantasies of wish fulfillment, positive or negative. It gives a heightened version of reality to fantasies of bliss as well as revenge taking place in reality, outer space, or an opium den.

Dialogues

Directions: "I am going to divide you up in pairs and give you a dialogue. One person will say: 'I'm leaving.' The other person will say, 'Don't go.' Each couple can develop the dialogue in their own way. We'll take them one at a time."

Discussion: Any short dialogue from our larder of time-worn conflicts can be used here: "I want it."—"You can't have it." "Yes, you did."—"No, I didn't." "Come here."—"I'm staying." "It's your fault."—"I had nothing to do with it." Even a simple round of dialogues starting with the word "Yes" from one person and answered "No" by the other can be used to set up further work.

Props

The director brings a variety of objects to the group—toys, articles of clothing, pots and pans, a mirror, a cane, an umbrella—any group of objects that might evoke memories or associations.

Directions: "Pick an object that draws you in some way. It could be something you like, or an object that reminds you of the past. Pick anything you have any feeling about. If two or three of you pick the same thing, that's fine. We'll take turns."

Discussion: After the objects have been selected, ask each person to speak as the object. (If the group is less functional, each person can just talk about the choice.)

These objects can be used in many different ways. Here are two more:

Different Uses

Directions: "I'm going to pass one of these objects around and see how many ways we can use it."

Discussion: The cane, for example, can be used to walk or dig with, as a sword, as a gun, to beat rugs, to threaten. This exercise promotes flexibility and imagination.

Commercials

Directions: "This time we're going to do something completely different with these objects. We're going to pick one, and then we're going to use it to make a commercial. Each one of you will have a chance to make a commercial for your prop. For example, you could us this little wallet to advertise your store. 'We have purses and wallets of the very finest quality. This leather came from sheep that roamed the highest mountains in China, so it's rough and tough and will last you for years. Buy a wallet like this, and you'll never choose plastic again.' " This warm-up enlivens the group and can be used to help cope with feelings of inadequacy in public situations, performance anxiety, or on the positive side, fantasies of commercial success.

Story Telling

Directions: "We're going to tell a story, one sentence at a time. We don't know where it's going. I'll start. 'Once upon a time there was a dark, dense forest . . . ' Now, Mary, it's your turn. Add a sentence. Anything you want. When we've gone all the way around the circle, we'll know whether the story's finished or whether we want to add more by another round."

Discussion: A quiet group often uses this warm-up to enter the imagination and begin to have fun together, while the director gains information about the group's tele.

Fortunately-Unfortunately

Directions: "I'll begin. Fortunately, I got here on time. Mary, you could continue with 'Unfortunately, you still had to start the group late (just an example).' Then each person starts with 'Fortunately, or unfortunately.' "

Discussion: Here is another warm-up that is an ice-breaker in a relatively high-functioning group. Teen-agers enjoy it a lot. It encourages breaking some verbal rules and teasing a bit.

I expect each member of the group to participate in the warm-up if at all possible. In very large groups, listening to each person would mean taking up so much time that the energy of the warm-up is lost. In groups of more than twelve to fifteen people, I try to structure a warm-up that can be done in small groups, or one that demands only a one-word or short-phrase response. The psycho-drama director must always try to find strategies that promote maximum participation. Some of mine follow.

I try to achieve a middle ground between utter spontaneity—which could result in one member's dominating the group and many others excluding themselves—and rigid directorial control, which can reduce spontaneity and create the feeling that group members must look to the director for every move. Thus, in relatively spontaneous groups, I often sit back and wait for individuals to respond as they feel ready. When the time-lag between participants increases, or when I see the group participation ebbing before all of the members have participated, I encourage those who haven't spoken to do so. In groups whose spontaneity is low, I ask a staff member (or anyone whom I can trust to cooperate) to begin, and then proceed around the circle. If an individual is reluctant to participate, I give support by structuring the task for her in more detail (see "Resistances and Some Ways of Dealing with Them," chapter 13) and then ask her to try it again. In case of an out-and out refusal, I ask the group member to listen to some of the other responses, telling her that I will come back to her at the end to see if she's changed her mind.

One of the warm-up's primary functions is to create an atmosphere of spontaneity and trust in a very short time. The exercises themselves present the group with a common bond. The director has to see to it that the process of warming up actually takes place; in other words, that the group members's responses are whole-hearted instead of mechanical. It is crucial to encourage or praise any contribution. The warm-up should provide a supportive atmosphere where an individual can take her first steps toward self-disclosure; it is helpful to thank each participant by a nod, smile, a short comment about her contribution, or a literal "thank you." A warm-up functions at its optimum when it gains momentum as it proceeds—group members join in more and more rapidly, respond to each other, relaxing their defensive formality or stiffness. Group members often expect to fail. *I don't know what she wants us to do. I'm not at all sure I understand what she said. Well, I'll try, but I probably won't get it right.* If the group director validates the sense of impending doom with a judgmental response, the group's spirit immediately sags and the momentum cannot build.

In the event that a group member actually misunderstands what is required for the warm-up, the director confronts a dilemma. She thinks: *I'd like to validate this response but how can I when it's wrong? The others will now become confused about what they're supposed to do. On the other hand, correcting this fellow in front of all these people isn't easy.* The group members, many of whom have noticed the misunderstanding, think: *Well, here it is. Just what I thought would happen to me. He made a fool of himself. What if she tells him? How humiliating. What if she doesn't? That wouldn't be right either.* My strategy for solving this dilemma involves two steps. First I validate his contribution. Let's say the warm-up involves speaking a few sentences John's therapist would say about him. John, however, addresses his therapist. My first response is "Thanks. Sounds like you have some pretty strong feelings about that guy." Then, having stuck to my dictum: "Never let a response go by without validation," I go on to the second step, which involves clarifying the warm-up for John. "Could you try one other thing? Play the role of your therapist, Dr. Rosen, and tell us about John. OK?" In order to be as clear as possible I may then repeat the direction to the next person. "Let's hear your therapist talking about you." With this strategy, I may be able to avoid the bogging down of the group that results from ignoring or downgrading the mistaken response.

A different sort of dilemma comes up for the director who has chosen the wrong warm-up. She observes her group's wooden responses, their lack of enthusiasm and discovers an undeniable lack of momentum. A freeze-out has replaced the warm-up. In that case, I change the warm-up. If I have any clue in the form of a small spark that momentarily flickered somewhere and then fizzled, I use it for my next attempt. If not, I may try something nonverbal, if the first warm-up was verbal, or anything that takes us in a radically different direction. Before making the change, I check my perception with the group. "Would you rather stick with this warm-up or try something else?" This gives me a chance to check on my own paranoia (there are times when the fizzle is inside me and the group chooses to continue with the task) and enables group members to be part of a decision to change course. The director's willingness to change has an additional advantage: it models spontaneity. It conveys the message: In this group you don't have to stick to anything rigidly. You can change to something more fun when you feel bogged down.

Since nonverbal warm-ups don't require participants to talk, they work well with groups of strangers or groups reluctant to open up. They are not resistance-proof. *This is silly. Like nursery school. Is it going to be one of those touchey-feeley California type games? I don't want to touch anybody in this group! I don't want to pantomime anything. That's like charades!* The nonverbal warm-up can be shared and reworked in psychodramatic terms. Nonverbal activities get people out of their chairs, but they have the disadvantage of requiring a transitional step before actual role-playing can start. Most of these tasks need to be followed by group discussion or verbal warm-ups to provide clues for further work. The discussion will be easier if there is room for silent reflection immediately following the nonverbal work. The director can say, "Let's take a few moments to get in touch with our feelings. What's going on inside you right now? Perhaps you're feeling an emotion. Perhaps you have some awareness of a part of your face or body. Just take a few moments to become aware of how you're feeling. Once you know, go back over the exercise. Did you notice any changes? At any particular place in the exercise? Take your time. It's OK if you can't answer all these questions. Anything you discover will help us work further." It is important to leave a three to five minute period of silence. The discussion can begin with questions like "What was that like for you? What was happening in your body during (after) the exercise? What part of your body are you most aware of? Do you have anything you want to say to any other member of the group? To me? Have you felt similarly in any other life situation?"

NONVERBAL WARM-UPS

Simple Movement

Some groups—groups of aging, or handicapped people, for example—have a difficult time beginning any complex activity, verbal or nonverbal. These groups can begin with simple motions. The exercise also works well with higher functioning groups who can use it for a variety of stretches to warm up, as long as there is no danger of the group's feeling infantilized.

Directions: "I'm going to begin with a simple motion and I want you each to copy me. Pass it along." (The director can lift a finger, scratch her ear, tap her foot, etc.).

Discussion: When the movement has been done by everyone, the director can enlarge the gesture, or change it, for several rounds. This exercise can also be done in unison, and, eventually, group members can take turns as director of the movement.

Rearranging the Room

(This applies especially where the room has been set up in a formal way-rows of chairs, chairs around tables, etc.)

Directions: "I would like to begin by changing the room around. We need space for a stage. And I want you to be comfortable. So make some decisions about how and where you want to sit—chairs, floor, table, next to whom—and where the stage could be. I would like you to work silently. If you need to communicate with someone, do it in pantomime." (Take five to ten minutes.)

Discussion: Recalling a child's setting up her play room, this warm-up usually creates an atmosphere of spontaneity. It can be used with groups of over twenty people, as choice increases with the size of the group. One caution: if the group members appear as stiff as the furnishings of the room, do not use this warm-up. It needs to be welcomed at least by a few of the group members. I usually follow up with one of the verbal childhood-memory exercises.

Walking

(This task is possible only in a room large enough to permit freedom of movement.) Both this technique and "stomping" come from movement therapy.

Directions: "I would like to start by moving around a little. So, I'd like you first of all to get out of your chairs." (It is always important to get the group to its feet as soon as possible—otherwise they will sit and listen.) "Get in touch with the space around you. Don't talk. Take a look at where you're standing, who's standing near you, who's far away." (Allow about two minutes.) "Now start to walk slowly around the room taking in everything and everyone with your eyes.

Don't talk and don't touch anyone if you can help it." (Allow two to five minutes.) "Now increase your speed and avoid eye contact. Walk faster." (Allow two to three minutes.) "If you are about to bump into someone, don't stop yourself—unless you really don't want to. Let yourself be jostled. Avoid eye contact." (Allow two minutes.) "Stop. Tune in to yourself for a minute to get in touch with your feelings. Notice any body sensations." (Allow 1 minute.) "Now walk slowly again, making eye contact, and let yourself make physical contact if you want to." (Allow two to five minutes.) "Good. Let's stop now and come back to the circle." This exercise can also be ended by saying, "I would now like you to find a partner (form groups of three, five, etc.)—still without talking—and stop when you've done so." At the end of a few minutes, check to see whether anyone is without a partner and help him find one. In groups where members do not know one another, this is an easy way to choose partners for further work.

Walking with different emotions and experiences: This warm-up can be extended by asking group members to walk according to different emotions.

Directions: "Now walk happily—sadly—You're angry. Surprised." Or try different experiences.

Directions: "Now walk toward someone and shake hands, like you've met an old friend. . . . Now walk home from a bad experience. . . . " The walk can be varied in speed, take up a lot of space, as little as possible, etc.

Discussion: I've often used this warm-up for day-long workshops. It is a good wake-up as well as warm-up exercise. It can be performed even by inhibited groups and has the advantage of being easy to do and yielding a lot of group contact and active movement.

The discussion afterward often centers around the experience of making eye contact, as well as other experiences about being touched or not touched by relative strangers, feelings about trust, intimacy, shyness and privacy and provides a natural bridge to further work.

Writing with the Unaccustomed Hand, a Movement-Therapy Technique

Some materials are necessary: paper, preferably large pieces which can be torn off a roll of butcher paper or from a large sketch pad, and crayons, charcoal, or pencils.

Directions: "Today I'd like to try something which most of you probably haven't tried before: Writing with your unaccustomed hand. If you're right-handed, that means your left—otherwise vice versa. Writing this way often helps you say something you feel and remember things you've forgotten. In order to get into it, I'd like you to imagine yourself when you were first learning to write. Where were you—at home, school, nursery school? Picture the details of your environment. If you learned at school, picture for yourself how you got there. Did you walk? What did the pavement look like? Did you drive? With whom? What was the building like? Did it have a particular smell? Picture yourself as you were then. How old were you? What did it feel like to be you then? You can close your eyes if you wish." I give these directions in a soft, unobtrusive voice so that I don't interfere with the group's concentration. Then I wait about five minutes, encouraging group members to stay with their fantasy and discouraging any talk. "When you feel ready, I'd like you to pick up a crayon and tear off a piece of paper to write on. Stay with your young self. You're probably five or six years old. Find a place to write—the floor, your chair, the table over there. Now, I'd like you to practice writing your name. If you had a nickname, maybe you could practice writing that."

At this point, I usually begin to take on a shade of the first grade teacher, supporting the group in their focus on an earlier time in their lives. After about five minutes, I continue: "Now, still with your unaccustomed hand, I'd like you to try writing a little story about yourself still as you are first learning to write. Tell us your name, how old you are, and anything else you want us to know. Don't think it out. Let it come through you. See if you can just let your hand do the writing, write what it tells you, try not to think it out." After people start to write, I notice the ones who are finished and discourage their comparing notes. "Let me know when you're finished by looking up at me, don't talk about what you wrote for now." When all but a few group members have finished, I say, "Those of you who aren't finished, why don't you just finish the sentence you're writing and then come back to the group?" Back in the group, I ask each person to read his story aloud, still in role.

Discussion: Like the verbal childhood memory exercise discussed earlier, this warm-up facilitates the recall of childhood experiences with surprising clarity. The work that follows can elaborate these memories by enacting specific situations suggested by the stories or by continuing with further childhood group activities. Once the task has been learned, it can be used for further warm-ups or continued group work. For example, group members can be encouraged to write letters to one another, to write about their families, to finish sentences in writing, always with the comment: "Try to let your hand do the writing for you."

Psychodrama is a way of playing. Writing with the unaccustomed hand is a direct route to the child in each of us. It never ceases to amaze me that a room full of worried-looking, self-conscious, wary "grown-ups" can so readily be transformed. Body postures and facial expressions change as memories bring back a part of childhood and then as group members warm to the difficult challenge of writing in this new-old way. People sit on the floor, sprawl, looking comfortable and absorbed. The stories are usually simple in language, very different from the way we usually talk. "I'm Cathy. I am five. I have a big brother and a big dog. I want to go to school but they won't let me." "My name is Bob. I like to run fast. School is lousy." "Dear Mary: I'm mad at you. You hurt my feelings. Goodbye forever. Love, Tom." In psychiatric wards, where the isolation of each client is almost palpable at times, writing with the unaccustomed hand often serves as a bridge between people. Our adult selves are experts at distancing others; as children we can reach out.

The Blind Walk, an Encounter Technique

Directions: After having people choose partners and pick the number 1 or 2, I say, "I would now like all the ones to close their eyes and the twos to lead them around this room. See how much rapport you can establish with your partner. Those of you who are leading can concentrate on giving your partner as full an experience of this environment as you can. You can touch, but don't talk at all." After five minutes, the procedure is repeated with partners reversing roles.

Discussion: The warm-up can end here with everyone coming back to the circle and, one pair at a time, talking with his partner about the experience. Because the activity requires a certain amount of trust, the verbal exchanges will reveal obstacles to intimate relationships. Further work can involve doubling and role-reversing and can then be expanded. For example, suppose Bob says to Tom, "I liked leading you but when you were leading me I tightened up, I just couldn't get myself to trust you."

Eva: Who else could you say that sentence to?

Bob: "When you were leading me I couldn't get myself to trust you?" . . . My wife, I guess. We're always arguing about how I have to be boss all the time.

Eva: Can you choose someone in the group to take the role of your wife? O.K. Start by saying the sentence to her, and Joan, just respond by fitting yourself into this situation.

The blind walk has many variations, some or all of which can be used in warm-ups. All should take five to ten minutes and be done by both partners in both roles. (1) "This time you can talk but not touch. Stay close to your partner and give him a verbal picture of what he is about to encounter, for example, 'You can take three steps forward, then you'll be close to a chair. Walk around the chair.' Adam, give your partner as full an experience as possible of this environment. I will be making some changes in the way the room is set up so that there will be some unfamiliarity for all of you." I then set up various obstacles: two rows of chairs back to back to make a narrow path, a stack of chairs as a tower, some overturned chairs, etc., changing these again as the partners change roles. (2) "Now I'd like you to try something very difficult. Talk but don't touch. I'd like you to keep a distance of at least three feet from your partner and I'd like the directors to encourage the followers to take risks. There's running, jumping, exploring new aspects of the room, skipping, etc. Keep your distance from your partner. I will be making some changes in the way the room is set up so that it will be unfamiliar in places." (3) "Both partners close their eyes. Touch but don't talk." (4) "Both partners close their eyes. Talk but don't touch." (5) "Shut your eyes and explore the room by yourself."

Blind walk variations two to five should be attempted only after one of the first two versions has been done. The last two can be anxiety-provoking and should be timed accordingly; two to three minutes may be enough.

If more than one version of these walks is done—as a prelude to a day-long workshop, for example—spontaneity and playfulness

increase with each task. If this doesn't happen and the group becomes more constrained, the warm-up can be discontinued and the
constraint used to stimulate further role-playing.

Family Sculptures, a Technique Developed by Virginia Satir

Directions: "I would like to try something new today. We haven't done
it before so no one knows how to do it. It's called family sculptures
and means that I want you to give us a living picture of your family.
Would you like to try it, John?" I pick John because he has indicated
conflicts with his mother and father in the last session. If the group
is very unspontaneous or new to me, I may ask a staff member to
volunteer, or I may sculpt my own parents, using members of the
group. If John agrees, I continue, "How many people are there in
your family? Could you pick someone to be your father, mother,
etc.? All right. Now I'd like you to sculpt these people into a picture
that would tell me something about the way your family relates. If
I were walking along in the park and saw your sculpture, what would
it look like? What picture would you get? Family members, your only
job is to be putty in John's hands. Don't talk, and let John mold
you into a sculpture. John, don't tell them how you want them to
look. Place them where you want them and mold their bodies into
the right position; you can even mold their facial expressions. Good.
Now put yourself into the sculpture." If John has difficulty understanding, some examples can be given. "You know, some people
sculpt their father with his back to the family and Mom and the
children huddling close together. Or you could put Dad down on
the floor with Mom standing over him, ruling the roost. There are
all kinds of possibilities."

After John has finished, I may ask him to give his sculpture a title,
and to take one last look around it to see whether he has achieved
his goal or whether he wants to add some final touches. Then I say
to the group members, "Be sure you each get a look at this sculpture.
If you can't see it from where you're sitting, come on over here and
take a look at each family member. Family members, hold your pose
for another minute or so, then you can relax."

Discussion: This warm-up opens up many possibilities. Each family
member can be asked to say a sentence that would fit the way he

or she felt in 'the sculpture. Group members may wish to speak for John, guessing how it might feel to be part of his family. Further work on John's family could follow, or a theme can be picked up from the group and tried out on various group members. In a group where the theme was isolation, several people had lines like, "I can't seem to touch or see anyone in this family." A theme can be pursued with each, asking whether the statement would fit for his own family and setting up a scene with family member(s) to whom he would like to say it.

Another way of working, especially if the group is scheduled for more than one hour, involves encouraging the rest of the group members to sculpt their families, reserving the decision about what to work on until the group has seen all the sculptures. If people are reluctant to sculpt their families, any other theme can be used for a sculpture: "Sculpt a person that you get along with in the group in the attitude you most like to see him. Sculpt one of the staff members in a way that really bugs you. Sculpt me in the way you see me operating in the group and then yourself in relation to me."

Sculpting is very rewarding. It accomplishes several goals: getting group members off their seats, permitting a nonthreatening form of touch, giving the sculptor a feeling of having some control in a situation—the family—in which he has often felt helpless. The sculpture also presents sculptor, family, and group members with rich themes for further work.

Nonverbal Conversations

Directions: After dividing the room in half, I ask the members to have a nonverbal conversation with someone on the other side of the room, using the way the conversation is going to decide whether to move closer or remain at a distance.

Discussion: Groups new to experiential techniques may be reluctant to engage in such an unusual activity. It should not be attempted with a new, shy group. Staff members can help to model the activity as it begins. This warm-up is very helpful when an ongoing group has been excessively verbal or intellectualizing. It provides welcome relief from an excess of verbiage and leads to a discussion in which nonverbal messages are the focus. The work that follows often has a more direct, vivid quality.

Machines

Both this and the next technique come to us from the theater.

Directions: After breaking up the group into teams of five, I ask each group to take a moment and assign the numbers 1, 2, 3, 4, or 5 to each member. I then pick a team to start the activity and say, "OK, now I'd like number 1 to come to the center of the room and begin a movement that could be part of a machine. Don't talk about it, just do it. Mystify us. You don't have to know what the machine is, just a mechanical movement. Fine. Now I'd like number two to come up and move in a way that relates to number one and makes sense in terms of creating a whole machine." I repeat the instructions for 3 and 4 and then ask 5, still without talking, to make sense of the machine and come up and show us how to use it. I will then ask him to tell us in words what the machine was and what he was doing.

Discussion: This warm-up tends to be successful in a group that has been "too serious" or unrelated—it is excellent for a group that needs to have fun and experience some spontaneous play. Further work will emerge from descriptions of the experience, associations to it, or fantasies aroused by the child-like quality of the task.

Nonverbal Gift-Giving

Directions: The group stands in a circle. "I'm going to give the person next to me a gift. I'm not going to talk and there aren't any real presents. I am going to show something about the quality of the gift by my gesture and how I hand it to him. He will then receive my gift and give a gift of his own to the next person." If further instruction is needed, I say, "Use your imagination. You can pick a rose from a rose bush and hand it to your partner, or take some sticky gum off your shoe—anything goes. You can put the rose behind your ear when you receive it, between your teeth or wear it as a corsage, you can grind the gum into the floor, throw it away, or stick it on your own sole."

Discussion: This warm-up is seldom appropriate for a new group. Nor would it work in a group where conflicts have arisen. But for a group already acquainted with each other and with nonverbal communication, it has all the delights that make gift-giving a natural occurrence.

The follow-up discussion usually produces poignant memories, which are easily used for further work, of other dreaded or welcomed gifts.

Stomping

Directions: The group stands in a circle. "We're going to try something really crazy today. First of all, I want you to stop talking and really get in touch with where and how you're standing. Get a little space around you. Get a good grip on the floor with your feet. Loosen your knees so you're free to move if you want to. Now, try stomping your feet. Stomp as hard as you can. Harder. If you want to make noise with it, go ahead. Are you worrying about the other people watching you? They aren't. They're either stomping or worrying themselves. See if you can forget everything but the stomping. Good."

Discussion: This exercise can only be performed if the people downstairs will put up with it. (We were once caught by an angry druggist whose pharmacy was right below us; he insisted that we had made several bottles jump from the shelves.) It cannot be used with individuals who might become overstimulated and lose control. It is valuable in bringing life back into a dead, tired group and encourages talk about the expression of aggressive, hostile behavior useful for further work.

Passing an Imaginary Object

Directions: "I have a ball in my hand. (Director mimes ball) and I'm going to throw it to someone in the circle. (Mimes throwing the ball.) Then that person will catch it and throw it to someone else." After the imaginary ball has been thrown to several group members,

I may add "Now the ball is going to change size. For one person it may be really really heavy, (demonstrates) for another, light as a feather." After the group has learned that they can transform the ball's size, they can transform the ball itself. "Now the person who receives the ball, can receive it as anything you can imagine—it could be a large gooey substance, or you might be catching a puppy—use your imagination."

Discussion: This is an activity for a relatively high-functioning group. It stimulates the imagination and usually works to infuse the group with playful energy.

Sound-Ball

Directions: "I'm going to make a sound and direct it to someone in the circle. That person will imitate my sound and then make a different sound of their own and direct that to someone else."

Discussion: Like the imaginary ball toss, this warm-up needs a flexible, spontaneous group. It can build energy and group cohesion and reveal a lot about group tele.

Rhythms

Directions: "I'm going to start with a simple beat (director claps a simple 1-2 beat) and I'm going to ask the person standing next to me to repeat it and add something. We'll go around the room until the last—poor person—is challenged to repeat the whole sequence."

Discussion: Here is another warm-up for a high-functioning or a musical group. It is energizing, helps to focus concentration, and can challenge a group to learn to listen and work together.

Handsqueeze

Groups are often difficult to close. An easy ritual that promotes group cohesiveness is the handsqueeze.

Directions: "Let's stand in a circle. Now take the hand of the person next to you. When we're ready, I'm going to squeeze the hand of one of the people next to me, I'm not going to tell you which, and that person will squeeze the person next to her and so on. When I get the squeeze back on my other hand, group will be over."

Discussion: If the squeeze doesn't come back in a reasonable amount of time, I find out where it got stuck and begin again. The activity can be extended by having others start the squeeze, by letting it travel quickly, by starting squeezes in both directions. It helps the group to leave with positive feelings.

Psychodrama demands that we play with children heavily burdened by their grown-up disguises. The atmosphere in our groups is usually rational, often serious, abstract, and wary. Self-conscious grown-ups fear the failures they were warned against by their parent grown-ups. The program calls for them to keep cool, calm, and collected; to know better; to think before they talk; to be mature; to do things right—stifling thoughts; thoughts which throttle spontaneity. The director, a clown in the circus of psychotherapy, uses the warm-up as a way of giving permission to be spontaneous. To flop, to be silly, to shout, to cry. To move around the room. To make noises. To remind the grown-ups that a child exists inside each of them.

4

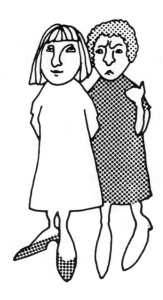

The Double

A technique originated by Moreno, the double is the most powerful single tool in my repertory. The double stands behind the protagonist with the intention of becoming a part of him so that she can voice something implicit in the scene, as though it were a new feeling or thought just then occurring to him. When she speaks, she must use the pronoun "I" and use masculine pronouns to describe his thoughts and feelings. She is not a separate player in the psychodrama. She must not forget that she is a part of the protagonist.

Before we begin to work with the double, I want to underline the importance of following, not leading. The double is an auxiliary, a helper with the specific job of finding a part of the protagonist that lies just below the surface. In order to achieve her goal, she must try to empty herself of her own reactions and open herself up to the protagonist. She must receive everything the protagonist offers as a cue to what he might be experiencing: his stance, his intonations, his slight shifts in position, his pauses, his sighs. Using all of these cues, she must also be sensitive to the protagonist's reaction to her contributions, so that she can work in a general range of potential acceptability. While she may want to challenge the protagonist at times, she never wants to lose him. She must stay in touch with the protagonist in order for him to experience her as a true inner voice, not another, different person standing behind him and giving her point of view.

Doubling is a unique method of communicating the nature of conflict and one of the most effective pathways for the expression of empathy. To double is to "put oneself in the other's place." John wants to work on why he is such a pushover with his boss. We ask him to confront his boss and find him timid and soft-spoken, easily ignored by his much more aggressive counterpart. We give him a double who—always within the boundaries of what is accepted by John—acts out his inner fury, shouts at the boss, threatens to quit— shows our protagonist in a dramatic fashion that there is another way to express himself. Tracking John's reactions, the double sees that he is somewhat taken aback initially, but quickly appreciates the rightness of his double's reactions. It takes very little time before John's own voice becomes stronger and he begins to represent him- self with a vigor that allows his double to then become a quiet, encouraging internal voice.

When I was a child I developed a game that probably began my doubling. Looking at pictures of old masters, I would assume the physical position and facial expression of persons in the painting. *If I were carrying a spear and my hands tensed to grasp it, my eyes wide open and eyebrows raised, what would I feel? Or, in my velvet gown, my hands idly playing with the lace on my blouse, my eyes cast down—what am I thinking about the man who is looking over my shoulder?*

Our language contains many phrases and metaphors expressing the essence of doubling: *If I were you . . . put yourself in my place . . . put yourself in my shoes.* We want to communicate our actions and our inner experiences. One of the most frustrating aspects of human existence is the fact that we can only express a small part of any experience—only the top of the iceberg shows. We've become so accustomed to our partial vision that often we're not even aware of the rest. The language is filled with a phrasebook of these frustra- tions: *Dr. Jekyll and Mr. Hyde . . . only a bird in a gilded cage . . . putting on a good face . . . still waters run deep . . . shallow brooks are noisy.* When we attempt to explore the inner life of another, we are often brought up short by conventions of superficial communication. *I know how you must feel . . . I've felt that way myself . . . I know . . . I've been there.* How do you know? How did you feel? Where have you been? Alas, the answers are available only in the rarest of circumstances. Doubling allows us a way to express the inner life.

To varying degrees, each of us is aware of conflicts, dualities, hypocrisies. Yet we often express only one side or one level of a given situation. Our culture places a premium on time, clarity, and lack of ambiguity. We try to say what we have to say clearly and briefly. We try to play unambiguously admirable roles. We are either brave or scared, moral or sinful, good or bad, angry or kind. We seem magically to believe that if we were to let in a conflicting feeling, or worse, to give it expression, all would be lost. Our culture labels feelings as potential harbingers of failure. *If I see someone caught in a fire, I can save him—but I mustn't remember that I'm afraid of fire, too. If I did, I might not be able to act, and if I were to say I'm scared, my chance to be heroic would be lost.* We often suppress emotions that could interfere with something we expect of ourselves. A good mother does not show frustration or anger. Men don't cry. We want to avoid becoming vulnerable. And so we hide tenderness or caring. *Play hard to get, stay cool, give him the cold shoulder.* The more important the hidden emotion, the more likely its suppression contributes to the development of symptoms. Doubling is a way to begin to give voice to the conflict within us.

The double is an inner voice. The voice of conflict, of self-pity, of irony. The double is the coward inside the hero, the saint inside the sinner, the needy child in the lonely eccentric. The double takes a chance on losing control by allowing tears, rage, tenderness. The double can raise her voice. The double can laugh.

Doubling presents endless possibilities and because of that, must be used cautiously. Doubling is not an avenue for the expression of one's own emotions unless they fit the person for whom one is doubling. The person who doubles must pay close attention to the cues given by the protagonist. She is there to help the protagonist become aware of conflictual feelings, to help him see alternative ways of expressing emotions. When the protagonist gives signs of rejecting the double and it becomes clear that what the double is saying is not relevant, the double must be flexible and let go of her precious hunch and try something else. (More of this in the section "The stubborn double.") I have observed that argument may not be a sign of rejection, however. An internal conflict is often expressed authentically by doubling. The surest sign that the double is doing poorly is when the protagonist makes no use of her contributions. She might as well not be there. She only takes up space. The director must give her a cue that leads to better understanding or replace her.

There is one other caution. Doubling is a powerful technique. When a double is successful, she is experienced by the protagonist as an inner voice, not as the other. For this reason, the protagonist often drops her normal defenses. If the protagonist were asked by her mother, for example, or even by a close friend, "Do you ever want to murder your husband?" she'd probably reject the notion out of hand, and tell us that, course she gets angry, like anyone else, but murder, ridiculous! If, on the other hand, our protagonist is confronting someone who role-plays her husband in a scene, and one of the usual endless arguments breaks out, and she hears her double saying, "I feel so frustrated I could kill you. I've thought of it before. I really could kill you," she may well agree with her double and then become frightened because of the intensity of her feeling. The double facilitates the expression of feelings which may be frightening and upsetting for the protagonist. It is important for the double to be aware of this possibility and to include it in her doubling so that, in addition to helping the protagonist to express feelings, she can support the protagonist in tolerating them. She may want to say, after our protagonist has agreed she could murder, "Now I've said it. And I'm really scared. I didn't think I was that kind of a person," or to ask "Did I scare myself? Did I go too far?" Or "Well, I said it, but I would never do it. But I sure feel it now and then! Wow!"

Both the group director and the double need to be aware of the protagonist's vulnerability. The double must carefully judge the protagonist's reactions to her doubling and be prepared either to comment on them or change the course of her doubling. The director must be prepared to find ways of giving the protagonist more control—to interrupt the scene, ask for the protagonist's feelings, send in another double with an opposite point of view, encourage the protagonist to argue with her doubles. Unless caution is observed, the risk is that the protagonist feels manipulated into saying something she wasn't ready to say.

New members of ongoing groups usually learn to double by watching others. Doubling is a natural technique and needs little explanation. In a new group, or with a new member of an ongoing group—let's call her Jane—I usually start by asking Jane whether she will accept a double. When she asks what that is, I try to be very brief in my reply, emphasizing that "doubling is a great deal easier to do than to explain," and that I'd like to ask Carol to double for Jane in order to say some of the things Jane may feel but not say. I may add some of the following sentences: "You know, you can argue with your double or you can agree. It's just the way it goes in our minds sometimes—two sides going at each other. If you feel your double is barking up the wrong tree, be sure to tell her so and tell her why. She may still keep going, but tell her anyhow." I have found the latter to be an important instruction because there often seems to be a misunderstanding on the part of the protagonist that the double is going to "tell the truth" about her. When the doubles are played by psychiatrists, nurses, or other mental health personnel, it is important for the protagonist to know that she does not have to accept what is being said, lest the doubling degenerate into a kind of mental health brainwashing.

I then make it clear that the rule is that only Jane can hear her doubles. Others in the scene with Jane cannot reply to what the doubles say. If Jane wants to say a sentence said by one of her doubles, she has to repeat it herself. This rule is very important because it (1) helps reduce confusion and (2) provides a way for Jane to take responsibility for herself and to make clear what she is willing to say at a given time. The confusion resulting from an argument of two people with their doubles may be overwhelming if all four voices can be answered.

Further, the double may be able to say something Jane can't and deprive Jane of an opportunity to say it herself. It may not happen in this scene. It will happen only if and when Jane feels strong enough to express her feeling but only Jane can decide when and how to take a stand. Jane is demure, while her double tells her husband that she's sick to death of him. Occasionally, by a victorious smile, Jane lets us know that her double is "right on." In order to face her hostile feelings, Jane will need to go one step further than to shyly acknowledge her double: she will have to say the words herself. On the other hand, Jane may not feel the hostile feelings her double attributes to her, or she may not be ready to face them. In that case, it is important for her to be able to talk to her double, telling her "But I'd never talk to my husband that way. He's been so good to me. Anyway, I don't talk that way," and have her double retreat for the time being.

I make one other rule in the beginning. The rule is that both the double and Jane always use the first person. If the double sees something Jane is doing and says, "You're twiddling your thumbs," she is no longer her double but a person outside of Jane, observing her. If she says, "I'm twiddling my thumbs," she can be perceived as a part of Jane, encouraging Jane to talk further. If Jane then answers, "No, you're wrong, I was scratching my other hand," she has again lengthened the distance between herself and her double, making her double the other "you," not the self. Even in such a seemingly minor disagreement, I insist that Jane keep using "I" as she talks with her double: "No, why would I twiddle my thumbs? I was just scratching my hand." It is very important to keep Jane and Carol from becoming adversaries. They're both Jane. Jane may have internal disagreements, questions. But she's asking herself, not somebody else. When the double is used correctly, Jane is hardly aware of her. She simply uses her to express her own feelings. In order for this to occur, the double must talk in such a way that she can be accepted by Jane. She can't talk simultaneously with Jane or anyone else because then Jane won't be able to hear her. She must listen closely to Jane in order to find the right times in which to speak.

If Jane agrees to let Carol double for her, I usually ask Carol to stand slightly to the side of and slightly behind Jane, and to assume a similar physical position. Carol needs to be near enough to Jane so that she can easily perceive Jane's physical reactions. Carol and Jane must not be face-to-face, since this position seems to enhance the feeling of oppositeness, of two separate people. When Carol, the double, is behind and slightly to the side of Jane, she can more easily be perceived as an inner voice. From Carol's point of view, the scene may go something like this:

Double: (*I'm Jane's double. Now what? How will I know what to do? I don't know what she's thinking. Jane's physical position tells me something about her. Let's see. She's sitting down. I'll sit down. She's crossed her legs; so will I. She's beating a tattoo on the floor with her left foot; I'm doing it. I feel impatient. Maybe that's what she feels. I'll give it a try.*) I'm feeling impatient. I want this to start.

Jane:	(*says nothing but nods her head in vigorous assent*).
Double:	(*This is the beginning. Now Jane and her husband are arguing. He is riding her about all the money she spends at the shrink's. What a bastard. That's how I feel but she's just sitting there. Tapping her foot again now. I know why she's impatient.*) I wish he'd stop talking. I'm so sick of this kind of talk. But I feel guilty, too. So I just sit here.
Jane:	(*ignoring double*) Well, what can I do? I really don't feel right about using the money you earn for my extravagances.
Double:	(*Oh, that Jane! No guts at all. I bet she's not feeling all that humble. Maybe I can goad her into speaking up for herself.*) I do feel right about using the money. I just haven't got the guts to say so. And I'm mad at him for bringing it up all the time. And I don't have the guts to say that either. (*Jane doesn't say anything. She looks like she might cry.*)
Double:	I'm almost crying because it's the same thing over and over again.
Jane:	It's true. I don't know what to do about it.
Double:	I'm sitting here the way I always do and you're talking on and on the way you always do and I want to tell you how I'm feeling for a change.
Jane:	Well, I do feel hurt because you seem to criticize me so much.
Double:	There, I said it. (*She isn't experiencing anger. She's hurt and she said so. She doesn't have that trapped, impatient look anymore. I like that. She seems more real now. They continue the scene. Jane practices saying something of what she's been feeling. Her husband hears her. I am needed a lot less as the scene finishes. I feel satisfied with how it went.*)

SOME STYLES OF DOUBLING

The Neutral Double

This double resembles the non-directive talk therapist. The double is there to understand the protagonist, to validate what she has to

say by putting it just a bit more strongly, and to give her opportunities
to look at different choices, mostly by asking questions.

Florence: I want to keep staying at my parents' house and they
                want me there too.
Double: They really do like it when I'm there.
Florence: Yes, they make such a fuss you'd think I was still in my
                teens.
Double: Sometimes I feel like I'm still in my teens when I stay
                with them.
Florence: It's true. It's hard to feel grown up in the house where
                you were a kid.
Double: Have I felt like a kid lately?
Florence: Yes (*pause*).
Double: How do they make me feel like a kid?
Florence: It's not their fault, it's just the way it is. Mom always
                watched over everybody and she still does.
Double: Good old Mom. Always watching. Does it bug me some
                of the time?
Florence: Yes, but there's no point in telling her.

The double does not emerge as a vivid aspect of Florence's personality. Rather, this double blends in with Florence, leading a bit here
and there, but always strictly within the framework of Florence's
words. If the double has a hunch about something that Florence is
not saying, she waits until Florence almost says it and then asks a
question. If Florence disagrees, the double will drop the argument.
This is of course the most supportive—and, at the same time, the
least dramatic—use of doubling. A client who has difficulty accepting
what another person says about him or one who is frightened that
the double will be able to "read his mind" will have the least difficulty
with this type of doubling. Anyone not used to having a double or
a protagonist who is showing signs of anxiety can be reassured by
these techniques. The client who flatly denies the double's statements
and uses them to fall out of role ("That isn't right, that isn't what
I think at all") can work more successfully with a neutral double
than with other types of doubling. When the protagonist expresses
confusion or helplessness, the double can switch to the neutral,
supportive role.

The Humorous Double

This double—well suited to my own style—is rendered effective by a quality that often deadens a psychodrama: the colorless, flat quality of the protagonist. The humorous double can exaggerate Florence's slow, quiet way of talking in order to get her to see what she is doing. Style is very important here. Humor always requires a light touch. The double must have enough sensitivity to stop and adopt a more serious style when necessary. She has to be at ease with her own sense of humor before she can use it therapeutically. If she inhibits what she's doing because she thinks Florence will be hurt or embarrassed, Florence will sense her inhibition. They will get stymied. On the other hand, she may be comfortable enough to go ahead, knowing that Florence might be taken aback at first but in the hope that she will be accepted momentarily.

Florence: There's not any point in telling my mom that it bugs me when she waits up for me all hours of the night. She'd still do it.

Double: There's no point in telling mom anything.

Florence: Well, I wouldn't want to hurt her feelings.

Double: I'm a very good girl. I don't hurt people's feelings.

Florence: It's true. I've just never been the kind of person who could just speak up and say anything.

Double: I'm too good.

Florence: I don't mean it that way.

Double: I don't even have any bad thoughts. At least not about my mother.

Florence: Oh, shut up!

Double: She's really getting to me now! I'm going to see if I can get out of this. But what if I hurt my double's feelings?

Florence: No, I'm not worrying about that. (*Laughs.*)

Double: What do I want to say to my mom about the other night?

Florence: I'd like her to just leave me alone more. Let me come and go as I wish.

The humorous double uses exaggeration in a good-natured attempt to bring emotions or defenses into awareness. John says, "I don't think I could even talk to my wife about this." His double says, "I'd probably disappear," or "I'm really weak" (slumping in his chair in an attitude of total weakness), or "My God! I might get angry and then she might get angry and then what?"

Mary complains about her loneliness. Her double may say, "No one else has ever felt like this. This is really unique. Because this is the kind of loneliness you can't do anything about." Or, "I certainly wasn't going to call anybody to talk about this. That would have spoiled it."

John says, "I've given up telling my kids what to do. They're over eighteen. They're on their own." His double says, "Now I just tell them how I expect them to run their lives. I don't tell them what to do. Just Dan about watching what he eats—he's overweight—and I want John to work with me, and I don't think Jane is ready to get married. That's all."

The most important aspect of humorous doubling is the double's willingness to be flexible. The double must know when to stop. The director can assist by encouraging John to fight with his double if he doesn't like what he's saying or ask John whether he understands the group's laughter and, if not, to ask what it was about, etc. When successful, this double often stimulates change. *It's hard to continue doing the same thing seriously once you've laughed at yourself in public. You're in this group where they're all supposed to be serious about their problems and everybody's laughing. Maybe it's not so bad as all that.*

The Empassioned Double

Psychodrama helps express feeling. Often, the protagonist's intense, passionate emotion is betrayed by her tension, body posture, or the tremor in her voice. But she can't express what she feels. Her voice remains quiet, her words colorless, her body posture rigid. The double, on the other hand, is free to express strong feeling. The double may exaggerate in order to show the protagonist a way to come out of hiding, to express emotion through language and the body. The cautions are many. The double's personal feelings about expressing strong emotion are important. *If I can't tolerate the expression of strong emotion myself, I'll be pretending or overacting and I'll distance, rather than teach. . . . I don't want to become so wound up in my portrayal that I forget that I'm doubling for someone else.* The double must continually check with the protagonist and use any opportunity that may help the protagonist express the emotion herself.

Florence:	I'd like my mother to leave me alone more. Let me come and go as I wish.
Double:	I want her off my back! I'm sick of being watched!
Florence:	She doesn't mean it that way.
Double:	I know she doesn't mean it that way but I feel it that way. Christ, why do I have to worry about her all the time! She does what she wants to do.
Florence:	I'd like to tell her to stop being so nosy.
Double:	I'd like to tell her I'm sick of it. But I'm afraid.
Florence:	Why am I so scared to get mad at her?
Double:	Why? Why? It's easier to think about that than to get mad at her, that's for sure. And I am really angry. (*Yelling.*) I'm sick and tired of being treated like a little kid!
Florence:	(*breaking out of the scene and looking at the director*) I wish I could talk that way. (*Laughs.*)

At this point, the director must pay close attention to the double and the protagonist. She may ask Florence to pick someone to play the role of her mother. (If this process looks like it may take long enough to break the dramatic tension, the director may wish to pick someone to play Florence's mother.)

The director says, "Here's your mother, Florence. How about trying to say some of the stuff that's hard for you to say. Use whatever your double said that fits and say it to your mother."

The double also stays in the scene and continues to model strong emotional responses for Florence. The rule that only Florence can hear her double helps encourage Florence to become bolder.

The empassioned double reduces conflicts to their bare essentials. John wants to talk about the "relationship" between himself and his wife. Jack, doubling for him, tells her: "You don't love me," or "I've hated you for years," or "I'm jealous of the kids," or "I love you and I want you and I think you're going to leave me."

Jane tells her husband, "Our trouble is that we don't communicate." Mary doubles for her and says: "You haven't talked to me about anything but business in fifteen years," or "I can't stand your silence another day. Sometimes I think I'll scream just to get some noise into the house!" or "I don't even think you know who I am anymore. You and the boys and fishing, me and the girls and PTA, and money. That's all we talk about. Who are you?"

John says, "I think we've drifted apart." His double Jack says, "I don't think you want me to touch you anymore," or "You're cold with me. I'm scared of you."

Jane says, "I think we've drifted apart." Mary, her double, says, "You don't see me as a woman anymore. I'm the lady that talks to you at breakfast and dinner and keeps your house and your children clean. I want you to hold me."

Mother says, "My children are members of the new generation. I don't understand them." Her double says: "I've failed with them. They're all crazy and they'll come to no good." Or, "They don't appreciate me. After all I've done for them. And now I'm all alone and they don't care." Or, "I'm furious with those kids. They use the house, my money, my car. And I let them. I'd like to throw those leeches out, them and all their friends."

Love. Anger. Tenderness. Self-pity. Protectiveness. Fear of death. Fear. So often, strong emotions become the subtext of a superficially banal conversation; they are betrayed only by a gesture, a tightening of the body, a breath quickly drawn, an "inappropriate" tear. The double's role is to bring the subtext to the surface. The advantage is that John's and Mary's cues are easy to read. We want to be known. *If my double is on the right track, I'm rooting for her to keep it up. If she's wrong, I tell her right away or I don't respond or I get bored. But it feels really good when she's saying something I need to say.*

The greatest obstacle to teaching humorous and empassioned doubling is our culture's caution about being "emotional." People who are free enough, open enough, loud enough, and soft enough to express strong emotions are hard to find. Those who judge the latter uncool, corny, or soap-operatic (depending on the age group) abound.

The Oppositional Double

Whenever our protagonist makes a suspiciously strong statement— especially when protesting too much—the double argues the opposite point just as vehemently.

Florence:	I hate my parents.
Double:	I love my parents, they take care of me.
Florence:	I'm tired of my boyfriend. I'm going to tell him I can't take his drinking anymore.
Double:	I love him. At least he lets me take care of him. No one else does.
Florence:	I'm not going to drink anymore. I know now that it's just stupid. I have to confront my problems.
Double:	I can't confront my problems. They're too terrible. I know I'll drink some more.

Sometimes this technique is used with two doubles:

Florence:	I don't know what I'll do when my mother-in-law arrives.
Double 1:	I'll tell her to leave.
Double 2:	I'll tell her to stay.
Florence:	I just can't face her. I'll leave a message with one of the kids.
Double 1:	That'll get her!
Double 2:	But what if I hurt her feelings and she gets upset?

These doubles intend to surprise Florence: to confront her with feelings which she has but does not usually admit to others or even herself, to show her alternatives, to entice her into conducting arguments she never thought possible. The director's job is to encourage Florence to argue with her double, lest the scene be one-sided and Florence simply let her double talk on without facing any of the conflicts implicit in her ambivalence.

Physicalizing the Double

Just as body language can be used as a way to gather information about how it feels to be the protagonist, the double's body language can show the protagonist another part of himself. Most often, the double gets her cues from the protagonist. If there is any inconsistency between what John, the protagonist, says and how his body looks, the double has a chance to dramatize his body language.

John:	(*sitting very stiffly, hardly moving a muscle in his face as he talks*) I like people. I always have. I'm easy-going.
Double:	(*mirroring and exaggerating the nonverbal cues*) I like people but I don't like them to come very close. I don't let them see very much of me.
John:	That's not true. I have very good friends.
Double:	(*in a monotone voice*) It's just that if I moved my face it might upset them. (*I know that John alternates between a show of great bravery and independence and total collapse—to the extent that he needs periodic hospitalization, and I use this information to make a point.*)
John:	I've learned a lot here and I think I'm going to be alright this time.
Double:	(*looking very weak, slouched down in the chair, speaking in a small voice*) But what about me? Who's going to take care of me when I get nervous?
John:	Come on, I'm not so nervous anymore.
Double:	(*leaning over and grasping John's hand*) I feel really helpless, somebody has to do something for me.
John:	(*undoing the double's hands, beginning to laugh*) Come on, take care of yourself, you baby.
Double:	But I'm the baby part of John. I need somebody (*clasping John's hand and sliding onto the floor, hanging on to him in an obvious attempt to drag him down*).
John:	Look, you can stand up on your own two feet. (*He disentangles himself and looks around the group, helpless, exasperated, amused.*)

Group members and the director team up to encourage him to fight the double, who has started to drag him down again. The struggle continues. John wins. John's physical victory over his double is cheered by the group. This is one instance where I do not insist that both double and protagonist use the form "I." It is clear that the double is playing a specific part of John, a part with which John is in great conflict. If this conflict takes the "I'm trying to get rid of you" form, it is realistic enough. There is no doubt that John is struggling with a part of himself.

I do not suggest using this type of doubling with inexperienced group members. John needs to trust his double. If he loses, he hears his double saying, "I guess I'm not so strong after all. I can't even get this double of mine on his feet." Winning isn't easy because the double can be just as stubborn as he is. The struggle is outrageously theatrical. Both double and protagonist have to be willing to risk appearing ludicrous. The goal is to anchor the message in John's body. Once he has actually struggled with this helpless part of himself it's harder to forget it, or to forget that he is strong. If John is depressed, engaging him in this battle is an almost certain temporary cure. *It's hard to stay depressed when your blood's rushing through your head, your breath is coming fast, and the crowd is cheering you on to victory.* This is an exercise in trust. John must accept his double as representing a part of himself—that is necessary for any doubling—but he must also trust his double not to hurt him or let him get out of control.

The Double as Counselor

Often, psychodrama grants a magic wish: "If I only could have thought then what I think now. If I only could have told him that then. Psychodrama gives the protagonist a chance to take time out, right in the middle of an argument. Florence and Fred are going at it:

Florence:	You do this to me one more time and I'm leaving.
Fred:	You don't mean you'd leave me over a little thing like coming home late because I had to work overtime?
Florence:	Oh no you don't! I'm not going to get caught arguing with you again. You know it isn't the first time! We've argued about this over and over again.
Florence's double:	There I go, caught right in the argument I wanted to avoid.
Director:	Florence, why don't you take some time out with your double to think about what you want to do next. Maybe you two could walk around together, talking about this situation. Fred, could you just wait while they do this? I'll give you and your double a chance to do the same later.
Florence:	It's true, I always say I'm not going to argue and then I do.

Double:	What do I really want?
Florence:	I want him to apologize.
Double:	That's what I want him to do, what do I want?
Florence:	I want him to see I'm right.
Double:	What do I want? What am I feeling?
Florence:	I feel so hurt and I wish he could see that.
Double:	Could I tell him that?

At this point the director asks Florence to talk to Fred again, starting the scene on a new level.

The main objective of the double as counselor is to disentangle the protagonist from the repetitive game, from winning or losing since, chances are, both mean losing. The counselor's hope is that Florence will become aware of the pain which underlies the quick repartee. The counselor-double lets Florence know she can take time out, that real feelings can be stated, that the same old argument can change and become productive.

The Collective Double

There are many times—the best times in psychodrama—when the group becomes a true audience, following each moment as though each one of them was playing a role. As director, I can see they are taking sides. In the center of the room, Joan is accusing her husband, Hal, of being unwilling to respond to her emotionally. She is crying. I look at the other people in the group, totaling about 25. Many of the men are showing physical signs of anger. Teeth are clenched, jaws set, fists clenched. The women on the other hand, look frustrated and outraged. Some are raising their brows in an exasperated expression and looking at each other and nodding in sympathy. Joan just can't seem to get her point across, but they understand. They've been there. When the scene between Joan and Hal has gone as far as it can go, one of my options is to let the group join in a "collective double." I usually begin by commenting on what I've observed.

Director:	I can see a lot of strong reactions here. You are feeling for Joan or for Hal. People seemed really involved in what Joan and Hal were doing. For now, I don't want

you to talk about what you were feeling. Instead, I'd like you to put yourself in Joan or Hal's place. As Joan or Hal, what would you like to say right now? Start by saying who you are and then say what you feel needs saying. "I'm Joan and I just don't know what's happening," for example. People usually join in easily. "I'm Joan and it seems so obvious that I have to show all the emotion in this family." . . . "I'm Joan and I'd like to get you into a good argument because at least it would show you're alive." . . . "I'm Hal and I'm tired of your nagging" . . . "I'm Hal and I can't do anything right."

Some men begin to take the woman's part and vice versa. John says, "I'm Joan and I really feel stuck. I'm doing the best I can and everyone is down on me." Mary says, "I'm Hal and I'm afraid. I'm really angry and if I let that stuff out I don't know what I'd do."

While the group is doubling, I assess Joan's and Hal's ability to listen. If the scene has left them frustrated and confused, and if either one of them is the kind of person whose confusion quickly builds to a paranoid feeling (*None of them understand, they're all against me*), I may want to limit the time of the collective double, or I may want to add some controls for Hal and Joan. Before we begin, I may tell them that I'd like them to just listen to the others for awhile, but if listening becomes difficult to let us know. I may simply ask them to comment if I notice a strong reaction. Or I may make a rule that Hal or Joan say a sentence in response to each of their doubles. If that is the choice, a voice from the group is always followed by Hal or Joan. Hal and Joan can express their reactions as they occur and the overwhelming cumulative effect of a dozen different Joans and Hals is avoided.

If Hal and Joan seem to me to be able to tolerate the ambiguity and confusion arising from the collective double, I ask them not to comment while the doubling is going on, just to listen. The group can then let off steam, building on each other's comments to say many of the things that they have held back both during the scene and with their own spouses.

When the doubling is over, there are several options. If Hal and Joan have not been talking, I ask them to do so. They need to express some of the feelings they've held back during the collective double—a one-way conversation always builds up frustration in the listener. I want to know what it was like to have so many doubles. If I find out that it was upsetting, I'll want to work now on Hal or Joan's feelings of being misunderstood by the group. If I find out that it was interesting or exciting, I'll want to know what Hal or Joan learned, what or who particularly touched them. I may then want to go back to working with Hal and Joan, starting a new dialogue with a sentence that Hal learned from the collective double.

I often use the collective double as a way of arriving at some closure after a difficult scene. No matter how ill-matched the people, how tenaciously stubborn the fighters, how well-rehearsed the conflicts, the group's expectation of a psychodrama is that there will be a resolution and "they will live happily ever after." (More about this in "Closure," chapter 16.) However, in actuality, an enactment often ends in an impasse. Hal and Joan continue the game ad infinitum; he is strong and silent, she rants and raves, neither gives an inch. The frog remains a frog and the princess a princess. The group is frustrated and disappointed. In the collective double, group members have a chance to vent frustration without directing it against Hal and Joan or the group. John may be inclined to say, "Joan, why don't you lay off him? All you ever do is pick fights." This would nail us tightly into the middle of the blame frame; Joan would feel attacked and attack back and the hopelessness of the discussion would pervade the room. If on the other hand, John says, "I'm Hal and I just feel so attacked by Joan, I don't know what to do," the content is the same but Joan is not being attacked; instead Hal is being invited to deal with his feelings. John may be inclined to say, "This group isn't helping. They aren't getting any better." Obviously, this is a tempting pathway for venting frustrations: It isn't that I'm not working at changing, it's that the group isn't helping me. If John says instead, "I'm Hal and I feel like nothing's changing. We're just doing the same thing over and over again," the problem of responsibility for change is laid on Hal's own shoulders, where it belongs. The collective double serves to clear the air. Group members have a chance to say what they've been storing up. Once the feelings are out, there's less need to blame or to insist on magic solutions. We are free to experience each other as people embroiled in complicated interactions occurring on many levels. We've each of us felt some of what Hal and Joan are stuck with. It isn't easy.

The Stubborn Double

All methods of doubling can be used by the same person during the same scene—consecutively, interchangeably, what you will—and all of them can be botched by the stubborn double. Nothing is worse than the double who cannot take no for an answer.

Florence:	I'm sorry to see them leave.
Double:	I'm angry at them.
Florence:	I'm not angry at them. I'll miss them.
Double:	I'm really angry at them.
Florence:	I don't know, I just don't feel angry at them.
Double:	I still feel angry, really angry.
	(*Etc., etc.*)

Obviously, this scene can go on forever. If the double is insensitive to the protagonist, she may become a sort of psychological saleslady, putting pressure on Florence, who either does not have or is not ready to face the feelings her double attributes to her.

The double does not lead. She is there to help the protagonist become more aware of her feelings, and help her see alternative choices. The double must never force her own individuality on the protagonist. She takes her cues from the protagonist. Florence could play her role in the scene without the double. The double could not be in the role without Florence.

Doubling for Florence I am filled with questions: *How would I feel if I were Florence? There. I said how I'd feel. Is she accepting it? No? Should I give it one more try? Was it a bored lack of acceptance or a passionate denial? If it's the latter, I think I'll give it one more try. Is she tensing up? Is she aware of it? Am I making her uncomfortable? Too much so to keep working? Can I be quiet and see where she takes this scene for a little while? Can I wait for her to give me the next cue?* The more questions I ask, the more material I gather for doubling, the less stubborn I'll be.

DOUBLING AS AN ADJUNCT TO THERAPY

Because doubling is one of the most flexible instruments of psychodrama, its use is easily extended to therapy. I have used doubling during sessions of both family and individual therapy. I use it most frequently for one of two reasons: either because someone is not talking, or because he's talking too glibly. In the first case, my questions are answered with silence; in the second, I find myself wishing for a quiet moment. In both instances, continuing to talk seems to make matters worse.

I had been seeing the Jones family for several weeks without making any headway with their fourteen-year-old daughter, Julie. While the rest of the family talked about problems they had with each other, or tried to talk about their problems with Julie to me, Julie just sat. She seemed alert and sensitive, but questions directed to her were usually answered with a sullen shrug of the shoulders—at most, a quick "yes" or "no." Needless to say, the family had originally come in because of their concern with Julie, who had got into a conflict with her parents over drugs.

For one of our sessions, the father had brought in a tape recording of Julie when she was allegedly on drugs and stated that he wished to play it for me. His tone was so judgmental that I had the feeling that if I cooperated with him, Julie would never open her mouth. I moved over to sit near her and said, "Julie, I have a hunch you want to say something to your dad about playing the tape." Julie, of course, shrugged her shoulders disdainfully. I continued, "Maybe we could do it together. I'd like to think out loud with you about the tape, first. I'll just be another part of you, OK?" Julie looked puzzled but didn't object.

"Let's see, I'm Julie," I said, beginning to double, "and Dad really brought the tape! I didn't think he'd go through with it. Wow! I am really mad. Doesn't he know I have feelings?"

Julie's eyes brightened a little.

I was concerned about Julie's father. Would he see me as taking his daughter's side against him? So far, he looked interested. I continued, "I'm really upset and when I'm upset I just can't talk. Especially not to them."

Julie nodded her head in surprise.

"Which doesn't mean I don't have anything to say. I really do want to talk to Dad about bringing that tape, don't I?"

Julie nodded again, more vigorously.

Here's my chance, I thought to myself. "Could I take a chance on saying it even if he doesn't understand it? Just to get it off my own chest? What do I want to say to Dad?" There was a long pause; Julie looked at me; I gave her an encouraging look.

"You shouldn't have brought that tape, Dad."

Julie began to vent some of her anger. At last, the silent treatment was over. Dad moralized in response, telling Julie he had made and brought the tape for her own good.

Again, I doubled for Julie, "See, talking doesn't do any good. I tell him I'm upset and he doesn't even hear me. He just goes on in the same old way. Why should I tell him anything? I don't think he knows I'm upset, even."

Julie nodded her head vigorously.

I made another attempt to get her unstuck. "Could I ask him if he has any idea what I'm upset about?"

Julie agreed and let her dad know that he was humiliating her.

Dad acknowledged her embarrassment. A beginning was made. During further sessions with the family, I used doubling not only with Julie, but for the parents as well.

Doubling enabled me to get out of the "teenager versus grownups" game and show my empathy for Julie without either patronizing her or validating her symptoms. In talking with the family later, I found that my fear of her dad's resentment had been groundless. He had suffered Julie's silences so long that any answer from her—even if it was negative in feeling and coming to him via the therapist—was a relief.

Doubling helps work with teenagers whose first reactions to therapy reflect their rebellious relationships to authority. Asked the usual questions ("What brings you here? . . . How are you feeling about that? . . . What can I do to help? . . . Could you tell me more about that?"), the teenager often responds with stubborn silence, or answers contemptuously. He is well rehearsed in these routines; doubling throws him off. Surprisingly, the teenager who refused to answer "How are you feeling?" often begins to respond when faced with a therapist double, who, sitting beside and a little behind him, says, "I feel terrible. Why did I have to come?" Teenagers are not the only subgroups likely to respond to therapy with recalcitrance. The person of a different race, the prisoner—anyone who feels that the system's cards are stacked against him—will respond more easily to indirect techniques.

My next example comes from individual therapy. During the few months I had been seeing Steven, each of us had changed how we saw the other. To begin with, I viewed him as an unusually literate, articulate young man, cleverly setting intellectual traps for me. There were subtle allusions, tests of memory, tests of my ability to tolerate his liberal views. I had passed with flying colors and we had spent the first few weeks sharing a delightful excitement. He was a smart client, I was a smart therapist; we were well matched and enjoyed jockeying for position. To my chagrin, this phase lasted longer than I had expected. Steven was reluctant to enter the realm of feelings. The closest we could get to his blocking of emotion was to talk about the trap. He knew that even when he wanted tell me something he was afraid of, he found himself blocked by distrust not only of me, but also of his own ability to recount the incident truthfully. There were traps within traps. Talking about this process wasn't enough; Steven continued dry and aloof, unable to get in touch with what I suspected were overwhelming feelings of loneliness and despair.

As we talked about his difficulties with his whiny, self-abnegating, mousy mother, it was obvious that he understood her problems and his own reactions to them—and that understanding wasn't enough. His talk was devoid of feelings. I began to sense a kind of sneering contempt in his intellectualization and began to double.

Eva:	If I'm you, I'm really bored with telling this story. I've told it to shrinks before. It never does any good, right?
Steven:	(*laughs*) Right.
Eva:	I'm sick of my mother's whining and I'm sick of my own whining.
Steven:	I don't whine. (*Steven objects strongly; I let him know by a nod of my head that I hear him.*)
Eva:	I don't whine like she does, thank God for that. But I'm sick of talking about things. About her. It never does any good.
Steven:	That's for sure.
Eva:	I feel strongly about her but I don't show it.
Steven:	I don't know what I feel. (*His mouth gets a stubborn look.*)
Eva:	I really hate her.
Steven:	It's true. I remember going into her bedroom and taking one of her favorite scarves and stuffing it in the garbage

can. (*Finally, Steven is in touch with his feelings. He is speaking with a great deal of vehemence now.*)

Doubling proved to be one of the only pathways to emotion. For the rest of the hour, Steven was in touch with a part of himself he had locked away: the hate-filled little boy, afraid to talk back to his mother for fear of hurting her, yet filled with rage at her selfishness, her self-destructiveness, her weaknesses. We could now see some of the roots of his own lifelessness and his continuing fear of asserting his anger, especially with women.

Doubling can be the heart of psychodrama. These vignettes represent some of its uses in various settings.

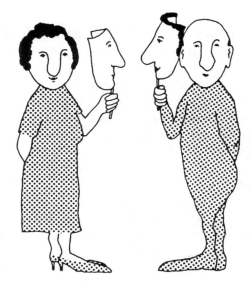

5

Role Reversal

Role-reversal is one of the quickest and most direct ways to learn about a protagonist's cast of characters. When the director talks with the protagonist to clarify what he wants to work on, his role-reversal with important others will demonstrate the roles for the auxiliaries. If John wants to work on his inability to confront his father's criticism, the director can ask John to be his father for a moment. Talking with John in the role of his father will acquaint the group with the kind of man and the type of criticism that John is facing. When a new person is brought into the enactment, the director can role-reverse John again and follow the same procedure.

Role-reversal also plays a major role during the enactment itself, or as an adjunct to therapy. We all play defensive games. When the conversation begins to feel risky, when we feel vulnerable we take a stance: we act the injured party, we counterattack, we distract, we show physical signs of distress, we lecture. The defensive stance can take any number of forms; but once taken, the conversation bogs down and what follows becomes repetitive and predictable.

John wants to tell Mary that he has been invited to be the speaker at his next business meeting. Mary, who feels that John has been drifting away and becoming more and more involved professionally, hears a threat and defends herself with a sarcastic "Well, there goes another weekend. Maybe I should write to your secretary and find out when you have a free evening." John's response is to withdraw by starting to read the newspaper. They are now playing the marital game "You Don't Love Me" and the chance to glow over John's business success is lost. What follows has happened many times. Mary's challenge becomes more and more bitingly sarcastic. John says nothing, pretending to be absorbed in the newspaper. She runs to the bedroom sobbing. He wads up the newspaper, throws it to the ground and then stomps out of the house, making sure the door slams loud enough to be heard by Mary. Early the next morning they reconcile without talking about the night so that the game can be put in storage just as it is, unaltered, ready for next time.

The beginning of a defensive game is a good time to begin role reversal: John and Mary are seeing me for marital counseling. I answer Mary's sarcastic response with "I'd like you to change roles for a moment. Mary, change seats with John. You're John now. John, you're Mary."

The participants must actually exchange seats. If the couple is to avoid confusion when both go back to being themselves again, they must literally change places now. If this is John and Mary's first role-reversal, I may take a little time to warm them up. I will address Mary (who is sitting in John's chair, ready to play John) "Let's see, as John, tell me how you're feeling about things as you begin this conversation with Mary. You've just had some good news, is the right?"

Mary:	(*bitterly*) That's right. I'm a big wheel at work.
Eva:	What kind of big wheel are you, John?
Mary:	Well, I get the most commissions in the place. I know how to sell. So I get higher pay and the bosses think I'm great. (*Mary laughs.*) It's really different at home!
Eva:	Is there anything you want to tell Mary, over here, about that? What's different at home?
Mary:	Well, Mary, you don't ever seem to think anything I do is right. (*Mary is still smiling self-consciously.*)

Eva: Go ahead, Mary, how about responding to that?

John: Well, all you care about is your work. That's all you care about. That's why you're gone all the time. I'm going to get a job as your secretary so I can see you every once in a while. (*John, too, is smiling as he does Mary's part of the familiar routine.*)

Mary: (*more serious*) Well . . . you just blame me all the time. How can I show you anything? I get so mad at you!

John is visibly relieved watching Mary describe his trap. If, in the original interchange, John could actually comment on what he's feeling instead of counterattacking or withdrawing, the game would not continue in the old way. Mary, playing his role, has shown him how to comment on his feelings. He could say, "I get so mad at you," instead of hiding behind the newspaper. I asked John and Mary to reverse roles again. "O.K., how about changing chairs again and going back to being yourselves? John, could you start with the last sentence Mary said in your place: 'Well, if you blame me all the time, how can I show you anything? I get so mad at you!' " When the director asks the participants to repeat the last sentence she makes sure that the scene will continue at a crucial point with the roles clearly assigned. Instead of thinking: *Let's see, now I'm back to being myself again, what did she just say to me? Should I start this? Or should I wait until she says something?* John simply says the sentence given to him by the director.

The director can follow any role reversal by asking the participants to comment. "John, how did you feel about Mary's portrayal of you? Could you tell her what you liked and didn't like?" I like to use role reversals where they can help the couple shift to a more useful way of talking. I leave talking about the role-playing for the end of the scene. Talking about what happened always lessens the dramatic flow. Only with a resistant couple that needs a lot of help from me in order to reverse roles at all, might I stop after the first reversal, in the hope that talking would provide encouragement. John may comment, "When you played me, you were really right on about my feeling hurt. How did you know I felt that way?" or "I don't think I talk like you did, I don't feel angry when that happens. I feel more hurt. . . . " We can then continue. The first comment may lead to an exploration of how Mary disguises her understanding of John's feelings: she's afraid to confront him directly because he would be upset if he knew she knew, etc. Further scenes can be done to discover ways for Mary to talk to John more directly. In the second instance, John can show Mary how he sees himself acting in the same situation.

Individuals new to role reversal may react negatively. "I don't think I'm like that. You're just being mean. You don't understand me at all." If Mary feels like this, she needs a chance to say so because she won't be able to continue in the enactment if she feels victimized by it. The director can then attempt to clarify the communication between John and Mary. Was John "goading" Mary by his portrayal and adding a new twist to the old game? Or was he simply trying to show her something he perceived about her? When the issues are clarified and we are, once again, outside the territory of the old routine, the role-playing can be resumed. Or, the director may want to adopt a different strategy altogether and help Mary out of her dilemma by further role-playing:

Director:	Mary, you're saying that John didn't talk the way you do. Is that right?
Mary:	Yes. I don't say things like 'I'm going home to mother.' He's just making fun of me. I haven't seen my mother in years.
Director:	What would you have said at this point in the conversation?
Mary:	Well, I guess I'd say, 'I'm fed up to here. Really fed up.'
Director:	O.K., John, could you say that line?
John:	I'm fed up to here.
Director:	Mary, is that more like you'd say it?
Mary:	It is. That's what I'd say.
Director:	O.K., then maybe we can go back to the scene now. Mary, be John again and respond to what he just said.

With this strategy, we can avoid the blameful discussion about John and Mary's conflict and give Mary more control where she fears ridicule.

Role reversal works well in any hierarchical grouping. In most places I work, there are staff members and clients. In some, there are students and teachers. Wherever clearly drawn roles exist-parents and children, teacher and student, supervisor and intern, visitors and inmates, employers and employees—one or several psychodrama sessions can center on role reversal. A warm-up on a psychiatric ward, for example, may involve my asking each person to choose someone about whom he has had some strong feelings: "If you are a client, choose a staff member; if you are staff, choose someone who is a client here." After giving the group adequate time for making a considered choice, I ask each group member to play the role of the other person and say one or two sentences about himself. For example, John is a client and picks Dr. K., about whom he has had strong feelings. He is now to play Dr. K. saying one or two sentences about John: "John just isn't getting anywhere. He just sits and won't talk," for example. I usually listen to each group member and then use a short feedback session to set up further scenes in which the staff-client relationship is reversed. In institutions with ongoing relationships, role reversal can be used to explore a recent conflict. New rules about room inspection were explored with house matrons and young women living in a girls' home with ease and good humor once a role reversal had taken place. In groups accustomed to using this technique, participants often ask for it: "I had a real set-to with Jane about coming here today, I'd like to try reversing roles and working on it."

For the director interested in working on parent-child conflicts, the following warm-up can be used to explore physical disparity. The group is divided into couples. Each couple is asked to decide who will be parent, who will be child, how old the child is, and a conflict. For example, a five-year-old might be refusing to eat his meals while a sixteen-year-old might challenge his father's rules about the use of the family car. One prop is necessary; each couple needs one chair.

The director then asks the couples to begin role playing their conflicts with the parent sitting on the chair and the child on the floor. After a few minutes, during which the director has made sure that each couple has found a conflict that can be prolonged for awhile, the director asks the parent to stand up and continue the conflict. For the first series, the child remains sitting while the parent first sits on the chair, then stands up, then stands on the chair. The same roles and the same scene are continued throughout all of these changes. The second series of movements involves the parent's sitting on the floor while the child first sits on the chair, then stands up, then stands on the chair, still continuing the same conflict. While this is not a complete role reversal, the exercise permits both players to experience the conflict from the reverse vantage point. The couples are asked to conclude the interaction by choosing a conclusion and enacting it at the same level.

This is a warm-up which is usually joined with enthusiasm, noise and excitement. (If the director needs a demonstration of this exercise, she can ask one couple to show it to the whole group.) Group discussions following the exercise usually center on power struggles: "I couldn't give any orders, I just felt more and more helpless the higher I got." . . . "I really liked being on top. Being small was awful. It reminded me of when I was little." . . . "When the child was standing on the chair and I was on the floor, that was perfect. Just like I feel at home. Like the kids are giants." . . . "I liked being level. That's the best way to talk, no matter who you're talking to." If time permits and the group is still interested, the whole exercise can be repeated with reversed roles.

For an excellent discussion of role-reversal, see Adam Blatner's* *Acting-In: Practical Applications of Psychodramatic Methods* (New York: Springer Publishing, 1988).

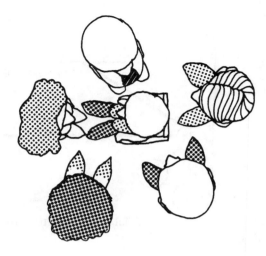

6

The Sociogram

The social sciences gave us this map of the protagonist's terrain, it enables us to learn about how the individual relates to his family, his job situation, his friends, whatever group has significance in his life. In sociology—I often begin my description of a sociogram this way when I am working with a group—the sociogram is a pictorial representation of an individual in relation to his group. We all remember having seen diagrams depicting John's popularity among his peers. John, represented by a circle with the J inside, has one close friend, Tommy, represented by the circle immediately next to his. He has three other friends, less close—children who live in his neighborhood he sees occasionally after school: Mary, Ted, and Jack. He feels isolated from the rest of his classmates and even more so from the other children in his neighborhood. A graphic representation of his situation might look like this: (see figure 4.1)

Anyone who sees this picture can make some guesses about John's life. He may be a member of a minority group—social, intellectual, or racial. His isolation may be based on a trait he shares with his friend Tommy, for example.

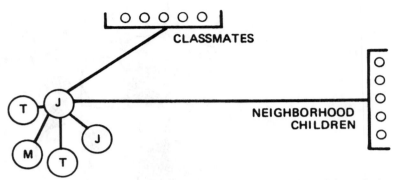

FIGURE 4.1 A pictorial representation of an individual in relation to his group.

The psychodramatic sociogram is a living picture. Instead of being represented by a circle on a piece of paper, John actually sits or stands in the center of his sociogram, assigning others in the group to roles and positions fitting significant relationships.

As the director of the group, I may want to use the sociogram to find out more about John's family relationships. If he is new to the group, I may begin with an explanation and follow by asking John whether he might like to explore his family relationships using this technique. If he is willing, the next step involves asking him to put his chair—or himself, standing—in the center of the circle; I often go there with him so that he does not experience stage fright. I then ask John to name the most important members of his family, past and present. He may want to include someone who has died; if the person was important at one time, he will continue to live in his psyche. As John names his family members, I ask him to find group members to take the roles of these individuals. Tele operates with invisible bonds that often supply just the right individuals—people who have some uncanny resemblance to the role they are playing.

If John is a member of a lower functioning group such as a psychiatric population, it may be difficult for him to cast group members: he can find no one who resembles his mother in any way, for example. If this occurs, the director can give him support by validating the impossibility of anyone's really taking the place of his mother: "I know there isn't anyone here who has just those unique qualities that make your mother the person she is. What I want you to do is to choose someone who might be able to play the role, to approximate some part of her." It is important for the director to avoid designating group members to play roles. Tele will help John intuitively choose individuals with the right qualities; no one else can know what these are. After John has assigned a role, I ask him to place the role player in relationship to himself in space—as close or as far away as the relationship requires. I also ask him to begin to role-reverse by demonstrating a typical posture for the role the player is taking. He may place the person playing his mother standing over him, or sitting with her back turned in a resigned or dominant posture, for example. John then chooses the distance and position of the role-players himself rather than passively accepting the way they choose to stand. After John has assigned a place and position to each of the significant family members, the first part of the sociogram is complete. We can now see a living picture of John and his family.

The second part of the sociogram involves assigning words and action to the living picture by using role-reversal. My instructions to John begin with asking him to think of one sentence for each person that is typical of the way that person might talk to him. A problem sometimes arises because John may understand that he is to find the sentence which shows the other person's attitude towards him. Therefore, the instructions must be clear: "Think of a sentence you might hear from this person. Just any of the things he usually says when you get together." The director accepts any sentence the protagonist offers. In my experience, responses range from a simple "Hi" to "What is your reason for existence, my boy?" As director, I know that deeper emotional involvement will emerge as we work further; all I need now is a start. After John has given each person his sentence, I ask the role players to commit it to memory so that they can say it when the time comes. After John has given all of them a sentence, my instructions to the role players are: "Now I want you each, in the order that John called you up here, to say your sentence to him. John won't answer you this time around, he'll just listen so that he can see how you are playing your role." I help the role players by nodding to them as their turn to speak comes up. After each person has said his sentence, I ask John, "How did they do? Look around the group once. Is there anyone whom you could help say the sentence more like the real person?" If John has suggestions for changes in the role playing ("My father would say that in a more aggressive tone," for example), I usually discourage further description of the differences and ask John to role-reverse to show how his father would say the line.

The third and final part of the sociogram allows John to interact with each of the role players. My instructions are, "I'm going to ask you each to say your sentence again, and this time I'm going to ask John to answer you. Then I want you to have a short conversation with John, continuing in your role. I know you don't know exactly what your character would say—there's no way you could—so I'm going to ask you to just follow your intuition, and continue talking with John until I stop you." Again, I usually give a cue that starts the dialogue with the person John called up first. As I observe the dialogue, I may want to help the participants reach a level of greater emotional depth by doubling for the protagonist or giving a specific structure to the dialogue, such as asking John to focus on telling the other person exactly what he is feeling. Often, however, no interventions are needed. A short exchange between John and each family member provides all the information we need in order to get a feeling for the relationship:

> *Mother:*   (*saying sentence assigned by John*) When did you get home last night?
>
> *John:*   About 10:30.
>
> *Mother:*   I was worried about you. I wished you had phoned to tell me when you'd be home.
>
> *John:*   I'm sorry.
>
> *Wife:*   Are they helping you at the Day Treatment Center?
>
> *John:*   I think the pills are making me worse.
>
> *Wife:*   I do too, why don't you stop taking them?
>
> *John:*   I probably should, but they tell me to take them.
>
> *Wife:*   Are you feeling any better?
>
> *John:*   No, I'm sorry.
>
> *Brother:*   You're going to be alright, John. Just stick to eating right and getting some exercise.
>
> *John:*   Thank you, George.
>
> *Brother:*   Have you tried going for some long walks; that always helps me when I'm nervous. Of course I never get as bad as you get.
>
> *John:*   I've tried it. Thanks for suggesting it.

In each dialogue, John plays a passive, receptive role. As we watch him, we wonder whether he doesn't feel any resentment toward all those fine people who are watching him so closely and trying to help him at every turn. We may want to explore this hunch by giving him a double who can make these feelings explicit. If John accepts the double ("It's true. I just wish they'd shut up and leave me alone some of the time. They seem to think I'm not trying"), our next step is clear. We can complete a part of the work with him by replaying the original scenes, this time with an effort on John's part to confront his negative feelings.

After the dialogues have been completed, the director and the other group members choose the enactments they would like to see explored further.

The sociogram provides a simple structure for getting acquainted with a new group or new group members. The step-by-step directions offer supportive contact with the director. Group members usually enjoy being chosen to play roles in the protagonist's sociogram. Since the protagonist does not have to do much talking during the initial phases of the sociogram, he can participate at a more gradual pace than an enactment would allow.

My work on psychiatric wards often leads to contact with individuals whose severe stress levels leave them withdrawn and uncommunicative. The sociogram offers a safe means of getting acquainted. A sociogram with an adolescent, for example, served to break the ice with a foster child who appeared suspicious and said only a few words during the warm-up. Assigning a sentence to each family member, he gave the same word to each person: "Hi." When I encouraged him say a little more, he seemed not to understand and repeated that people just usually said "Hi" when they saw him. I had my doubts about the value of continuing with so little information, but I sensed he was cooperating. He had chosen several people to play roles in his family; he was sitting in the center of the stage area. With a little patience perhaps something more could be learned. Then, as he answered each person (the reader will not be surprised to learn that he answered by saying "Hi" as well), a staff member noticed a growing tension in his body as he answered his mother. When I asked him about this, he answered that he had read his mother's "Hi" as a cross-examination about where he'd been and had stiffened defensively in response. With this information, I encouraged the woman playing the role of the mother to continue to pressure him, and found our reticent adolescent increasingly vocal and expansive.

The sociogram has been especially useful for a single consultation with a new group. After the warm-up, I ask one of the group members to do a sociogram of the group from his point of view. If the group is large, I may limit him to the six or seven individuals most important to him. He may see certain members as close, others far away; he may have a special place for the boss, etc. Often, after one sociogram is completed, other group members volunteer to do their own version and, after the initial work is done, I have in front of me a map of the crucial relationships in the group.

The sociogram has many uses outside of psychodrama. A family therapist may want to ask an individual to do a sociogram using his actual family members; a group leader may wish to ask someone to graph his social relationships in the group; the sociogram may include inhabitants of the same apartment house, friends, neighbors, shopkeepers—the sky's the limit. The technique's only requirement is time: I would not begin a sociogram unless I knew that I had thirty to forty-five minutes to work it through.

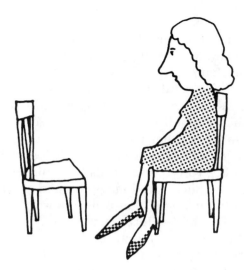

7

The Empty Chair

Originated by Moreno as an elaboration of role-reversal, this technique was later developed by Fritz Perls, the founder of Gestalt therapy and a regular at Moreno's Beacon Hill workshops. My own acquaintance with the empty chair stems from my personal encounter with Perls which taught me something about myself and acquainted me with a new technique and some of its specific applications.

Where others use role playing, Perls uses an empty chair. If a person, for example, wants to work on a problem involving his mother-in-law, Perls' response would be: "Put your mother-in-law in the empty chair and talk to her." John has showed the group he wants to work by sitting in the "hot seat," the seat next to Perls himself, opposite which the empty chair was located. I prefer to sit or stand next to the person who wishes to work, and place the empty chair directly opposite him. Here, where I can listen and observe nonverbal clues, I can show him that I am really listening and touch him reassuringly.

If John seems hesitant I may say: "Before you talk to your mother-in-law, why don't you tell us who you see there. Visualize her sitting on that chair. Tell us what you see."

It is useful to coach John so that he can give us the concrete physical details which help him visualize the person. "Well, let's see, she's about five-foot-five-inches, sort of dumpy, about sixty years old. One thing, her mouth is always going. She never stops yakking."

John has almost begun a dialogue; here is something he is upset with, expressed in words he could be saying directly to his mother-in-law. Such emotionally charged phrases provide the natural bridge to the dialogue that is to follow.

Now John addresses the empty chair: "Jeez, Mom, you just never shut up. Your mouth is always going. You never stop yakking. Yak, yak, yak" (turning to me) "but I'd never tell her that." I may make it clear to John at this point that we are interested in getting at his inner conflicts, that this is not a rehearsal, this is surplus reality.

I continue, saying, "Well, you just said it. Let's see how she reacts. Switch chairs. Be your mother-in-law and react to what John just said." As in any other role-reversal, John must actually switch chairs before continuing, to help him concretize his task and avoid the confusion that often results when several roles are played in the same location. John, playing his mother-in-law, now says, "Oh, I have never been so hurt! I don't believe it! After all I've done for you kids." From here on in, the director's task is to help John develop a dialogue that will help him express feelings he holds back in real life.

The dialogue may lead John to a new understanding of the conflict with his mother-in-law. For example, the director may notice that John instead of becoming angrier and angrier seems to lose vocal power, to become more and more the little boy as he addresses her. "You're always right, aren't you," John whines, "you make me sick. You don't even know what you're talking about."

The director may ask John, "How old do you feel?" If John acknowledges feeling like a boy, the next question is "As a boy, who would you be talking to like that? Who would you say that to?" (re-iterating the last phrase heard in the dialogue) " 'You make me sick. You don't even know what you're talking about.' " When John makes the connection to a more primary character in the drama of his own life, "It's true, that's just like my grandma that used to live with us and I'm acting like I did when I was seven," the empty chair now becomes Grandma.

Perls developed the empty chair as a way to avoid the deadening intellectualization of "talking about" problems and conflicts. It can also be used by the therapist in individual sessions because it facilitates the use of role-playing. In individual therapy, important others in the client's life can be brought into the hour almost as though they were actually present. Even in a talk therapy group, the empty chair may have advantages: unlike role-playing group members, it is always informed about the real situation and sensitive to the working individual. The empty chair can be used as a way to introduce group members to new characters in an individual's drama; the therapist may ask group members whether anyone feels he could now play the role of, for example, John's mother-in-law, after observing several exchanges with John playing the role in the empty chair.

So far, we have discussed the empty chair as a way to role-play others without using other role-players. The technique can also be used to act out symbols, metaphors, and dreams that help the individual get in touch with conflicts that represent inner struggles, fears, or anxieties not necessarily related to other people.

When I attended my first Perls seminar, I occupied the empty chair after so much hesitation that I was the last person in the seminar to work. Even after some initial work, I was aware only of my fear.

Perls:	Can you close your eyes and visualize your fear? Give it a landscape. Stay with your feeling of fear. What do you see?
Eva:	(*surprised that the images flow so readily*) I see an attic. Just a part of the attic with a brown wood floor. I can see the texture of the wide boards. It's dark and cold and at the very back of the attic, way back, there's a blue light.
Perls:	Could you talk for the floorboards. Be the floor. What does it say?
Eva:	I'm brown, and old, very worn. I'm dark. I'm cold. I'm really alone. No one ever comes here. (*I start to cry, experiencing a desolate loneliness.*) There are no people here at all.

Perls: Now go over to the empty chair and be the blue light.
Eva: (*changing chairs*) I'm way back of the attic. I'm light. I'm cold, too. I'm very beautiful, an icy blue. I can see my rays a short way through the window along the floor.
Perls: What do you have to say to the floorboards?
Eva: You're so dark and ugly. Why don't you come into the light?
Perls: Switch chairs and answer.
Eva: (*switching chairs*) Because I can't move. (*Again, I am conscious of great pain.*) I can't touch you. You have to come to me. (*I don't feel at all hopeful that this will happen.*)
Perls: Switch again.
Eva: I can't do anything about your feelings. I am where I am. You have to come to me.
Perls: Switch again. Now ask the light, "How can I touch you without being frozen out?"

Suddenly, I am flooded with the awareness that I have frozen others out of my life, coldly rejecting their warmth. The work put me in touch with my loneliness and also with the part of me that makes sure I stay that way. Perls has me say, "I can freeze you out" to several group members. I do it with conviction. My mood lightens. I tell Perls that I feel better. He asks me to shut my eyes again and to visualize my present mood.

Eva: Now I feel as though it's a warm day. I really feel warm. I feel like I'm just slightly underwater in a lake. And I can feel seaweed lightly brushing up against me.
Perls: Can you do that to some of the people in the group? Just lightly brush up against them?

I do. I lightly touch one person's hand, another's face, another's shoulder. I feel relieved. There's also a part of me that can connect with others. I feel that I want to be warmer. Maybe I can leave some of that coldness with the past, when I needed the self-protection it offered.

The empty chair can act out inanimate objects, dream figures, metaphors—roles difficult to cast with real persons because their inner significance is known only to their creator.

Perls believes that every aspect of a metaphor or dream is a projection. The dream that I am a grasshopper being devoured by a cat contains not only the fear of being toyed with, being eaten alive, but also my sadistic element, my devourer, the part of me that toys with others. The dialogue between the grasshopper and the cat puts me in touch with my weak-strong polarity, an inner conflict I need to resolve. A dream involving an empty parking lot slowly being filled with cars produced a dialogue in which the dreamer got in touch with his passive, blank way of resisting (the parking lot) and his more outgoing, aggressive drives (the cars).

A metaphor may be observed in an individual's posture. If I notice an individual's hand gesture, I may say, for example, "Could you take a look at what your hands are doing?" I may have to caution the individual not to change the position of his hands, just to observe them. The right hand is clenched. The left hand is covering it, the thumb making stroking movements. Right and left hands now enter a dialogue that demonstrates the individual's tension, anxiety, and anger. On the one hand (literally) his neediness, his want of comfort, love, and affection. If the individual does not remember dreams or show much in the way of nonverbal gestures, a meaningful metaphor can be elicited by asking the individual to close his eyes and visualize a given mood. Whatever emotion is experienced—fear, withdrawal, laughter, frustration, anger—this strategy involves asking the individual to "Visualize this mood. Close your eyes and see if you can go into your feeling. Give it a landscape. Give us pictorial details of the landscape your feeling calls up." Different elements of the emerging picture can then be placed on the empty chair.

The empty chair can be used during a family interview or psychodrama when someone who is absent or no longer alive takes on emotional importance. An empty chair can be used to represent that person. Now the others in the scene have to stop talking about the individual; they are directed to talk to him, as though he were once more among them. The strategy may involve having a member of the scene play the role of the absent member some of the time, or it may not. I am inclined to leave the chair empty throughout the scene—a symbol of the absent member, dead parent, divorced father, etc. Often the remarks addressed to the empty chair are messages for someone present, messages that have been diverted because of the convenient scapegoating of the absent member. With this strategy the director can take up unfinished grief situations—situations in which death or departure came suddenly, where the remaining members inhibited their feelings.

The empty chair is a bridge to the completion of unfinished emotional work, the investigation of metaphor and to direct emotional experience, for anyone that uses active techniques.

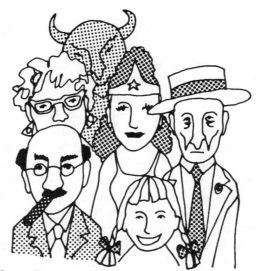

8

Six Characters in Search of a Personality

The six-character technique was adapted by Virginia Satir, who made many innovative contributions to the experiential therapies, especially family therapy. Although many techniques help us dramatize an individual's relationships, few exist solely for the purpose of exploring the inner life. This exercise takes us on an excursion into the soul.

The six-character technique requires a verbal and imaginative group and a leisurely pace. It will not work in a crisis. The directions are as follows: "I want you to think of six well-known characters, six famous creations—three men and three women. They can be from any age and any medium: book, play, movie, fairy tale, comic strip, television, advertisements, etc. They should be three men and three women who stood out in your imagination as you were growing up to be an adult."

The more literate and/or imaginatively spontaneous the client, the more easily he will respond to the task. Clients who have difficulty coming up with famous names often ask whether real people may be included. Because this exercise works best when the characters selected are larger-than-life—mythic, archetypal—I will allow real-life characters only as a last resort.

After the client has chosen six characters, he is asked to choose someone to play each role and to supply each role player with three adjectives describing his character. For example, one protagonist chose Captain Ahab and the Sphinx among his six characters. For Ahab, he gave the following three adjectives: "restless, driven, obsessed." For the Sphinx: "wise, elliptical, catlike." (I will describe his scene later in some detail.)

After all six characters have been chosen, the directions continue: "Now we are going to invite all six of your characters to a party where they will meet and talk. You will stay on the sidelines with me and watch." The director then directs each character to say his name as he joins the party. As in real life, there is a bit of awkwardness in the beginning, as the role players warm up to their roles. But, just as in an actual party where people need a little time to become acquainted, the ice is often broken after a bit of small talk. As the scene progresses, the group may become divided by antagonisms and coalitions which vividly represent the protagonist's inner conflicts. The director's job is to remain sensitive to the protagonist so that she can help him cope with the scene he has evoked. After ten minutes or so, the director may want to ask the protagonist to help the role-players by role reversing or suggesting changes in character or in the direction of the scene. If the scene becomes chaotic, or if an argument reaches an impasse, the director asks the protagonist to suggest ways of resolving the difficulty.

The length of the enactment is up to the director's discretion. When I feel that most of the conflicts and polarities have been explored, I usually stop the scene and ask the protagonist what he experienced as he watched. It is not unusual for him to respond by saying, "That's exactly what it's like for me all the time. That's me. That's the way I talk inside myself."

The director can explore the scene further by asking each of the players to give a monologue in which he describes his feelings while he played his character. The director can also ask the protagonist to do two things: (1) to say to each character in turn, "You are my . . . (tenderness, hatred, energy, etc.)," and (2) to arrange his six characters in a sculpture showing their relationship to each other (the humble Siddhartha may be on the bottom of a pyramid topped by the greedy Miser, for example) and then to fit himself into the sculpture in the end.

The six-character technique suggests topics for further exploration in the group. Does the individual like what he sees? Now that he has had a look at the party, are there any characters or scenes he wants to explore? The protagonist can pose questions, set up specific conflicts, impose monologues which let him know secret thoughts—in short, he can direct his characters to do whatever he wants. After he has seen his characters in action, he may want to explore his reactions with a double to help him integrate the experience.

AN EXAMPLE

Soon after I had learned the six-character technique, I became an enthusiastic proponent. The following is an example of its use in a group composed of young unmarried people who had been meeting together for two hours a week for about a year. The group had responded enthusiastically to the opportunity of acting roles which had such universal appeal. An ongoing joke in the group was that no one—including the therapist—could give up being "special," no matter what the cost. It was easier to find someone right for the part of Jesus Christ than for the role of a group member's mother who ran a grocery store in the Bronx.

Soon after the group began, Michael volunteered, asking to use the six-character technique. He had been giving it a good deal of thought, he said, and already had his characters in mind. Michael is a man in his early thirties, an architect known for his originality and his moodiness. He frequently wore an arrogant, aloof expression that made him difficult to approach. The other group members responded positively to his request. Perhaps this would be a chance to get to know him better.

I asked Michael to cast his six characters, to chat with each of them in order to find out how each saw the role he was assigned to play. I also asked him to fill them in on what he wanted in each character. I then asked Michael to give each person three adjectives that would describe the qualities of action he wanted.

Michael chose three men first. He asked the oldest member of the group, Robert, a highly gifted mathematician, to play Captain Ahab from Melville's *Moby Dick*, giving him the adjectives "restless, driven, obsessed." Robert knew and loved Moby Dick as well; there was an immediate understanding about what Michael wanted in the part.

Next, Michael asked Tad to play Siddhartha. Tad was a bit of a bohemian, a quiet young man with soulful eyes. He was not familiar with the Hesse book from which the character derived, but he had read a great deal about the Buddha in books dealing with Zen Buddhism and seemed to grasp what Michael wanted. His adjectives were "kind, quiet, responsive."

The next characters Michael chose were Pagliacci, from the opera about the sad, cuckolded clown, and Rima, the woodland sprite from Hudson's *Green Mansions*. Pagliacci was played by the group clown (of course), Larry, who portrayed a basic sadness while he made the rest of us laugh. Leah, playing Rima, was unfamiliar with Hudson's novel, but so right for the part that everyone knew she would have no difficulty playing the mysterious, attractive forest dweller. Michael selected June to play Ayn Rand—type-casting, they said in the group, for June was a powerful individual of considerable intensity in her manner. Her adjectives were similar to Ahab's—"restless, powerful, intense." Last, he asked Justine to play the Sphinx; her adjectives were "catlike, elliptical, wise."

The characters entered in the order of their selection. First, Captain Ahab. He looked gaunt, his facial expression even more tense and inward than usual. He introduced himself as he had been asked to do: "Captain Ahab." He gave a few short glances to his surroundings, apparently judged them lacking, and found a place near a window. During the rest of the scene, he looked out the window, making only short but powerful comments to the others at the party.

The Sphinx entered. She was a tall, wise-looking woman who conveyed a feline air. She looked about, a Mona Lisa smile on her face as she encountered Ahab's glance. "I am the Sphinx," she purred. (The group reacted with some surprise, Justine had not shown herself so seductive before.) Rima bounced in. She was young and pretty, dark ringlets cascading about her face. She had taken her shoes off. Her face was quiet and relaxed, yet she seemed to be smiling. She walked directly up to the Sphinx. "Hello, I'm Rima, a friend of Michael's. I've never seen you before. Do you know him well?" The Sphinx, who had made herself comfortable on a nearby sofa, said nothing for a while, apparently appraising Rima, who seemed to enjoy being looked over. Then the Sphinx said, "I know him better than he wishes me to."

As she was speaking, Tad entered, introducing himself as "Siddhartha." It was immediately apparent that he meant to talk to Rima. They were quickly involved in a conversation about the surrounding forest. The Sphinx looked on quietly; bemused, interested.

Ayn Rand came in. An older woman like the Sphinx, but her opposite in character. Restless, apparently aggressive, but without a target. She took to her part with obvious relish. (In the group, people often told June to slow down. Now she could be as quick and intense as she liked.) Ayn Rand paced the room. She thought that perhaps she and the Sphinx had met before at a writer's conference. When the Sphinx smiled "no," she attempted a conversation with Ahab, who also put her off, making it clear that he wished no connection with her. Ayn seemed surprised for a moment. It was difficult for her to believe that she was not the center of attention. She began to pace again, obviously hoping to break into the intense conversation between Rima and Siddhartha.

Pagliacci entered. He was appealing in his hippie attire, a sad look in his eye, apparently searching the room for someone who might understand him or show him some warmth. He introduced himself, then walked over to the Sphinx's sofa and sat cross-legged on the floor in front of it.

"I remember you," she said, "the last time I saw you I had to avoid you because I knew something you didn't know."

"I guess everybody knew but me," he countered sadly. "Maybe it was better that way."

"Surely," said the Sphinx. "But that was a few months ago. You're not still sad over that woman?"

"No," said Pagliacci sadly, "I'm much happier now."

The Sphinx looked around the room. "Happiness is like water," she said, "crystal clear in one moment and opaque the next."

On the other side of the stage area, Ayn Rand, addressing Siddhartha, said, "I really have no taste for these things; they seem so artificial to me. What do you think?" He had looked at her with some surprise because she had interrupted the silence he and Rima were enjoying. Now he turned to her, but before he could answer, she continued in a hasty, intense way, spewing out words in a torrent, "I know I've met you before. I said that to the lady over there and it didn't turn out to be true, although it still could be true as far as I'm concerned. People don't always remember. I usually do. But you, you. . . . Where did we meet? You look a great deal like a young man who used to work for me as a sort of secretary, but of course that wasn't you. Could you be related? His name was Gautama." (June was making an intellectual point here—obviously enjoying the response she elicited from some of the others who had caught the reference.) "An Indian fellow, so, of course, that wouldn't be you. But there is something so similar in quality. Something quiet about you, also, just waiting to be touched. I think I could help you find your creative energy. I think I could help you write. I have strong intuitions. . . . "

Siddhartha turned to look for Rima. She had gone to another window, at the opposite side of the room. He touched Ayn Rand's hand and looked at her quietly. "I don't know what you want," he said, "maybe I was related to that other person but he and I aren't the same. Excuse me, there is a man here I would like to meet." And he began to walk toward Ahab.

An awkward period ensued. The scene began to take on the appearance of a real party that was going badly. People didn't seem to know what they were there for. Some looked to the director for help but got only a quiet signal to continue. They milled about, saying a tentative word but making no real connections. On the outside of the circle, Michael was visibly disturbed by what he saw. He looked at me with a frustrated expression. I asked him what he was feeling.

"Like it isn't really happening," he said. "All these strong characters and yet none seems right for the others. They each seem to be in their own world."

I asked Michael what he would like to have happen between the characters. Michael responded that he would like them to make a stronger effort to relate to each other. I asked him to speak to his six characters, asking them to become more involved, less self-centered.

"Where have I heard that before," he said, looking back at the rest of the group, smiling in recognition of a message he had heard many times in his life.

On stage, the characters were eyeing each other. Ayn Rand, catching a glimpse of Rima who was crossing the room, said, "This party isn't going anywhere. Come talk to me. You are a very pretty girl. Pretty girls usually love parties like this. But you don't look like you are enjoying yourself at all. Why not?"

"I'm afraid of that man," Rima answered, indicating Ahab. "He frightens me. He's like a dark force. I want to be light and happy but I can't as long as he's around."

She looked at the Sphinx who had been sitting on the sofa nearby, "What do you think?"

The Sphinx smiled at Pagliacci, who was still sitting near her. "Why do we have to have fun? Joy and truth are seldom united. Maybe yes. Maybe no. But I don't care. Anything is alright with me."

"You have a poetic quality," said Ayn Rand to the Sphinx, looking deeply into her eyes. "You are a very unusual person. You have power. I'm interested in power. Are you sure we haven't met before?"

The Sphinx turned toward her. "I'm sure," she said.

Ayn Rand's eyes began to scan the room restlessly once more.

Offstage, Michael asked me if he could stop the scene in order to arrange a dialogue between Siddhartha and Ahab. I encouraged him to do so.

Ahab was standing at the same window he had chosen when he came in. His expression was somber, uninviting.

Siddhartha approached him. He asked, "Would you mind talking to me a little? I've been looking at you. Are you angry about something?"

Ahab turned to look at Siddhartha. He looked angry. He seemed to consider not answering the young man and then to think better of it. "I am angry," he said, "that all these people are twiddling their lives away." Siddhartha asked him what he meant. "There's nothing going on in any of their souls," Ahab answered, "They're like mush. No substance. No character. I am a very different person. I can't be expected to get along with the likes of you."

Siddhartha looked concerned. "But you are different," he said. "You look like a man who is driven by a great cause. What is it?"

When Ahab described his obsession with the white whale, the darkness that Rima had mentioned earlier became real. His face twitched as he spoke. At times one had the feeling one could see sparks flying, he was so intense. Everything else had been obliterated in his life; only Moby Dick existed. Clearly there was no room for human concerns in this fanatic's life. (The role suited Robert, often accused of an exclusive attachment to mathematics by others in his life.) And yet there was something attractive about his passion and his certainty. He knew. As we listened to him, we became aware that Michael, the protagonist, could be similarly uncompromising.

Siddhartha had listened quietly, looking on Ahab with patience and kindness. "I know you know I am not like you," he said when Ahab came to a stop. "And I know that you wouldn't listen to me if I asked you to think more of the others in your life, to be more compassionate. You are on a mission and you must live through it. It's too bad. I wish you could have seen me." He looked a little sad as he said the last words.

I had noticed Michael's growing involvement and had stepped close to give him support by my presence. Michael had tears in his eyes as the dialogue ended. He looked at me. "It's like me and my father," he said, "only I'm the intense one and he is kind and forgiving. But we never seem to be able to get together."

I asked Michael if there was anything further he wanted his characters to do. Michael thought it over and said, "No, I don't think so. I'm still shaken by that Ahab part of me. I think I'd like a little time to take it in."

A technique often used by Moreno is called the soliloquy, where the protagonist or auxiliary is asked to stop interacting with the others and, facing the audience, speak his thoughts. I felt that Michael's impasse might be a good place for him to explore and asked him to do so.

Michael (turning to the rest of the group). "Oh, that Ahab! I wish I didn't understand him so well. I'm the same way when I'm on some project. I just forget everybody else and I'll do anything to get it done, anything. I remember my mom used to come into my room when I was building models when I was just eight or nine years old and I'd just kick her out. Later she told me it really hurt her feelings but I didn't even notice. And I'm still the same way. I just have to learn to include someone else in. But I know myself. I just reach a point where everyone else is a big bother."

I thanked Michael and asked the group to take a five-minute breather. When we reconvened, I said to Michael, "I'd like you to do one more thing with your six characters. Tell each of them what quality of yours he represents. How would you feel about doing that now?"

Michael agreed and proceeded without difficulty. Naming the qualities seemed to help him finish, to settle something for himself.

To Ahab, he said: "You are my ruthlessness."

To Siddhartha: "You are my kindness."

To Pagliacci: "Oh, I'd forgotten all about you. You are my pathos."

To the Sphinx: "You are my wisdom."

To Rima: "You are my ideal."

To Ayn Rand: "You are my ruthlessness also. And my ambition."

Michael sighed deeply when he finished. He had been completely absorbed by the task. When we talked with him about what it had been like afterward, he seemed astounded. "There were so many familiar themes," he said, "but Ahab, he's the one that really got to me. What am I going to do with that part of me?"

I was pleased with the way the scene had gone. There were many themes we could return to: the polarity between the driving, obsessive demon and the love-starved young man, for example. When we reviewed the scene, Tom, who had played Pagliacci, commented that he had felt left out; everyone else had got more attention.

Another group member laughed, "Isn't that the story of your life, Michael, feeling left out?"

Michael joined in the laughter. "It's true. If I just didn't have to make such a federal case out of every little rejection."

I observed that Michael was relating easily. The scene had provided a much-needed bridge between him and the others.

Because the six-character technique requires a high-functioning group, I have not used it on the psychiatric ward; it would prove to be too great a challenge. In groups with a growth-oriented atmosphere—encounter groups, therapy groups—the six-character technique stimulates spontaneity and the use of the imagination. Eleanor Roosevelt, Elizabeth Taylor, Rima of *Green Mansions,* Jackie Kennedy, Alice in Wonderland, the Sphinx, Little Red Riding Hood, Marlene Dietrich, Ahab, Moses, Ulysses, Hiawatha, Linus of *Peanuts,* Siddhartha, The White Knight, St. Francis of Assisi, Bill Clinton—the cast of characters is unlimited and the potential for group enrichment immense.

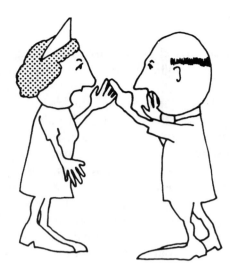

9

The Given Scene

Each new setting provides the psychodrama director with a number of opportunities. At a meeting of the Parent Teacher Association, relationships between parents, teachers, children, and issues relating to school can be explored. A given scene for a PTA meeting might be about a parent attempting to influence a teacher about a grade, or a scene where the parent or teacher is confronted by a child who refuses to obey, saying, "But my mother (teacher) lets me do it at home (school)." These scenes, which refer to issues common to all of the group members, are also called sociodrama. When the group and the director are new to each other, when there is a dearth of specific issues brought up by group members, or when the director needs to pull the group together, sociodrama dramatizes a common bond.

The answers to the following questions will help the director who is looking for a given scene: Who belongs to this group? Does the group have subgroupings which show potential conflicts (parents-children, parents-teachers, nurses-clients, etc.)? Does the purpose of the group announce common problem areas (Alcoholics Anonymous, psychiatric ward, therapy group, probation officer training group)? What kind of warm-up would help her discover the given scenes?

At a PTA meeting, the group can be asked to divide into pairs with one member of each pair assigned to the parent role and the other to the teacher role. If I have already discovered a common theme, I may ask each couple to work on it. For example: "Now that you have assigned roles, I want the parents to come in to talk to the teacher about the F Johnny got in math. You parents are upset about the F; you feel it will ruin Johnny's chances for getting into college. That is the only information I am giving you. The rest is up to you. Take a few minutes to decide how you wish to play the scene. Is Johnny capable of succeeding? Does the teacher wish to teach Johnny a lesson for being lazy? Are the parents overly ambitious? After you have decided, start your dialogues and continue until I tell you to stop. I will be coming around to listen to you." As I listen to the dialogues, I will decide whether one of the scenes might be useful for demonstration to the whole group, or whether we should ask each small group to show us a bit of their dialogue. We can then develop the scenes by asking the audience for different outcomes, to tap out one of the characters and continue the scene in a different way—in other words to explore in detail the most relevant aspects of the work.

On the psychiatric ward where I work, there are several given scenes: the scene of the client arriving at the hospital and talking to the admitting nurse; the scene of the client returning home from the hospital; the scene of the client asking the therapist whether she is ready to leave; the scene where the client tries to find a new job after leaving the hospital. In the next section, I will describe the course of such a given scene: the job interview.

THE JOB INTERVIEW

When I arrive to do my psychodrama group on the psychiatric ward of one of our large city hospitals, I learn that the clients discussed job interviews at the community meeting earlier in the day. Several unresolvable questions arose: Should you let a potential employer know about your hospitalization? Should you just omit it from your history? But then, how could you even talk about having been mentally ill?

I know from previous meetings that this group is lively, verbal, and intelligent. When my group begins, I decide to forego a warm-up (the community meeting warmed up the group already). "I hear you've been discussing the job scene. (General assent.) I'd like to do some more work on that if it's OK with you. Who is about to go out on a job interview?"

Shirley is a woman in her mid-thirties. She is nice-looking, neatly dressed, alert, energetic and tense. She volunteers that she has interviews with several employment counselors coming up that afternoon. She talks in the sing-song of her former profession: elementary school teacher. Another client volunteers to do the interviewing. (For once, I can take volunteers. We do not depend on tele to play the role. Sociodrama demands only that the role-player understands the generic qualities of the role.) In the opening scene, Shirley does very well. She states what she wants clearly—a job as a receptionist-typist—and looks out for her own interests in terms of time and money. She gives the impression of self-assured competence. Her hospitalization is not mentioned.

I get the feeling that Shirley and the client playing the interviewer are avoiding something. I ask, "Is there a question you're afraid the interviewer may ask, Shirley? "

She answers, "Yes. It's because I've only had this one other business experience, the job with the undertaker. Other than that I was a teacher and I don't want to go into that, because then he'll ask why I'm changing and all that. Anyway, I don't even want to mention the job with the undertaker because they might ask for a reference."

"And?"

"And my old boss knows I came here. . . . Well, I quit working for him in a sort of immature way. That is, really, I never quit. I came to the hospital and then I phoned him and told him I was here and I wouldn't be back."

Marilyn, an aggressive-looking younger woman who, on the surface, looks tougher than Shirley, nods her head, "I did the same thing." Several others comment that nothing is harder than to tell someone you're quitting.

We now have a common theme for more sociodramatic scenes. First, I ask Shirley, our undertaker's secretary, to phone her former employer to discuss her references. We play the scene with two outcomes. In the first, the employer is happy to help Shirley out by omitting her hospitalization from his references. Shirley thanks him but lets us know that she doesn't think it would work this way; in reality the scene would be different. The second time, Shirley coaches her employer in the role: he would feel morally obligated to let others know that she has mental problems; he would have to tell the truth, if asked. Again, Shirley astounds us with her firm, clear statement of what she wants. When she hears the bad news, she simply says, "Thank you, then I won't list you as a reference," and hangs up the phone. She is pleased with herself and tells us how different she feels from her earlier self, the woman who could not face quitting her job.

I believe that this is just a little too easy. Shirley comes off competent, all right—but the scene provides for so little exchange of feeling that we can't judge how easily her smooth surface might be ruffled. I ask her to do one other scene, the scene she avoided by coming to the hospital, where she confronts her boss and tells him she is quitting.

Now Shirley shows another self. Before the scene begins, she goes on and on telling us why she needed to quit the job: the pay was terrible, she had to get up at 5:00 in the morning for the commute, she had been promised a raise, he was impossible to talk with, etc., etc. But when she actually confronts him, she talks about herself, not the job: her inability to take pressure and tells him that her children need her when they come home from school. It's as though she expects him to feel sorry for her and fire her for her own good.

The group dubs her "the Mouse," and gives her advice on how to stand up for herself. Marilyn, the younger woman who seemed to identify with Shirley's problems earlier, shows Shirley how to be strong and tough.

Of course, I know that Shirley can't copy Marilyn. She would be pretending a toughness that is not her own. I take what might look like a step backward and ask Shirley to show us her real feelings toward her boss, tough or not tough, whatever they are.

She says, "I don't know why I'm here. I know I'm wrong to quit. You've been nice to put up with me. I know I'm just lucky to even have this job." She breaks up, laughing, "this crummy, dirty, cheap job, you bastard! OK, look, you know it's a crummy job so I guess

you can expect some turnover. I'm leaving at the end of the week."
Shirley laughs again as she talks with the group, more in touch with
a polarity inside her: the doormat versus the strong, free spirit.

Throughout Shirley's work, I have been conscious of Marilyn, who
has been acting as though she knew what to do, suggesting that
Shirley take action through unions and government agencies against
her funeral director boss, yet I remember that Marilyn had also
stated that she also had been unable to quit her job. When I ask
her about that, she agrees that she identifies with Shirley. Marilyn
wants to work on it. I ask her to play her boss, discussing Marilyn's
qualities as a worker:

"She was really good. The best I ever had here. Dependable.
Efficient. But then this crazy stuff. I just don't understand that at all."

What does he know about it, I ask.

"Nothing! Just one day she doesn't show up and then I get this
letter a week later. She says she wants to come back, just for an hour
or two to start with, and at first I thought it would be OK, but now
I don't know."

I ask Marilyn to choose someone to play her boss for a scene
where she talks to him about returning to work. She is obsequious.
"I liked working for you so much. . . . I always knew where I stood
with you and no other boss was ever like that. . . . Even if I can't start
again right away you should hire someone else, if there is ever a
time after that where you do need someone, would you give me
a call?"

Several group members point out to Marilyn that she seems to
be begging her boss to take her back, that she is saying: "Poor me,
hire me because you pity me." Someone in the group guesses that,
unlike Shirley, Marilyn doesn't want to work at all—that, actually,
she is talking herself out of a job rather than into one. One theme
pervades this session: "I can't decide whether I want work or pity
more."

This is a bright, sensitive group, and the members quickly find
out that Marilyn is deeply disappointed in her husband, who has
been at home for the past three months since he was released from
prison. In truth, she feels like a chump. She wanted her husband
to get a job.

As often happens with a given scene, we segue from the sociodramatic context to a psychodramatic one. (In a new group, such a

change would have to be carefully introduced.) One of the ex-convicts in the group plays Marilyn's husband, smoothly conning, "You know I've tried to get work, but who's going to hire an ex-con? . . . So I get up late, so would you if you had prison hours for a year. . . . If I didn't care for you and the kids, would I be here?"

Marilyn makes abortive attempts to show her husband the firm toughness she had voiced earlier but demonstrates again and again that she is unable to take a firm stand. We guess that coming to the hospital was her only way of saying she doesn't want to take care of her husband anymore. The group members point out to Marilyn that she presents such a tough, aggressive front to the outside world that it is hard to see her soft, helpless side. It is easy to see that others rely on her for help without thinking that she needs support herself. Just the day before, one of the group members had described her as hostile and distancing. But now she feels the group's support.

The examples show different ways of approaching the given scene, in this case, the job interview. In the first, we stick to the actual job situation, using the scene to finish unfinished business by investigating alternative solutions. The work with Shirley could have stayed in the sociodramatic mode and led to work with others who also wanted practice in the job interview. It would have been possible to work on a scene where someone who wants to discuss the fact that he has been hospitalized (or has been mentally ill, or in psychiatric treatment, etc.) does so and examines the consequences. In our group, the work led to a psychodramatic scene often explored in psychotic groups—the exploration of Marilyn's conflicts about work. Almost everyone in an all-day or overnight treatment setting worries about rejoining the outside world. Marilyn's words say "I want to work," but her real message is "Don't hire me." We could then do further work with the group on the more general issues relating to the need to appear strong while feeling very weak.

The given scene is also appropriate for a range of students, from high school to the graduate level, and can be used in many specific situations, for example, with women about to rejoin the work force after raising a family.

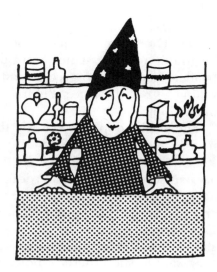

10

Magic Shop

Some techniques can be used as a warm-up, to fill up an hour, or to provide a whole day's work. Magic shop is one of these. At its best, it recalls the wisdom and spontaneity of fairy tales and children.

When I give the directions, I usually assume a tinge of the story-teller. My object is to weave a spell, to create an atmosphere of play, magic, daring, to establish metaphor as king, to encourage extravagant projection. I may use this technique because it's raining out and I need cheering up, or because everyone in the group seems to want to be someone else. Whatever the reason, when the magic shop takes hold, it usually takes up the rest of the session, however long. When it doesn't take hold, it's like any magic that fizzles—disappointing, tawdry, boring, and infuriating. This is a technique most useful for people in touch with their sense of serious play. I don't usually try it with strangers.

The directions: "The magic shop is a very special shop. You can get all kinds of things there for all kinds of prices. It has just one limitation: it only deals in human qualities. Oh, and one other thing. Magic shopkeepers aren't interested in money. Not at all. They only barter. One human quality for another human quality. Are you beginning to understand? You can get whatever human quality appeals to you—anger, greed, kindness, humor, humility—if you're willing to pay the price. Before you begin, you need to know one more thing.

The magic shop only exists in the imagination. It needs an imaginary location, the place you'd conjure up if you were to set up a store. We've had a store seven leagues under the sea run by an ancient sea serpent; a store set up in a clearing in the forest run by an age-old ageless shaman covered with leaves; stores in trees, on crags, in aeries. One shopkeeper was a spider who set up her shop in a corner of the cross of a medieval church in Cologne. If the shop has a clear location, it's easier for the clients to decide whether they want to shop there or not. And how to get there. The shaman in the forest had a hummingbird for a client, for example, who was bartering for relaxation. The spider was visited by a squirrel who couldn't be persuaded to give up any of her charm for the ability to express fury.

Let's start by imagining where you'd set up your shop. Close your eyes if you want to. Get a clear picture of the place. And of yourself in it. Where is your magic shop? What manner of shopkeeper are you?" I usually allow about three to five minutes. With these directions, everyone participates in the magic shop, and is better equipped for further work. Here is an example of what may follow:

Director:	Who's got a shop all ready to go? Could you tell us about it?
John:	The shop is in Muir Woods in an ancient redwood tree. Not in the tree but in the base, where a cave has been left by a fire near the roots.
Director:	And who are you?
John:	I'm a very cranky, irritable lizard. (*Group laughter. John is a somber staff member.*) But my shop is really full. I have everything everyone wants and a little more.

When the technique is used as a warm-up, the director may want to stop at this point and ask others about their shops, each of which is, of course, a metaphor for the shopkeeper's existence. As a warm-up, the technique quickly provides cohesion in a group familiar with the language of metaphor. If the director wishes to set up an enactment, he will continue:

Director: Would you like to set it up?

John: OK. (*A tree is fashioned from some chairs and pillows.*)

Director: How old a lizard are you?

John: Oh, I've been here since the fire, about 200 years ago, and I don't remember how old I was when I came.

Director: OK. You sound like a kind of scary storekeeper to me. But, there's probably someone here who wants to deal with you. People will go anywhere for a bargain. Who wants to go?

Mary: I do.

Director: Who are you and how are you going to find John's tree in the forest?

Mary: Can I just be me?

Director: It's better if you can use your imagination and find a shape and method of transportation that would fit this particular magic shop. Otherwise, how would you know about it?

Mary: Well, I go to this psychodrama group and . . . (*laughs*). OK, OK. Let's see . . . I'm a fawn. Just a little fawn traipsing through the forest. Everybody in the forest knows about the shop. So I'm just walking along.

Mary is a pretty, fawnlike creature. The audience is delighted with her choice. From here on in, the director's job is to see that active bargaining takes place. John is enjoying his role.

John: Good God! I hope I don't have any customers today! They're always messing things up. Urggg! (*Sticks his tongue out.*) I have a long sticky tongue. They'd better watch it. (*Disappears behind the pillows.*)

Mary: (*Having walked around the room a bit, she now pauses in front of the shop. Her voice is eager and friendly while the lizard remains terse and harsh except for momentary lapses.*) Knock, knock, anybody there?

John: I'm not going up there. This store isn't for children.

Mary:	Knock, knock. Anybody there?
John:	(*whispering and refusing to budge*) No.
Mary:	Hello there! I heard this is a magic shop. I want to trade with you.
John:	Oh, alright then, have it your way (*appearing with his head out from under the chair*). What is it you want? Make it fast.
Mary:	Well, I heard you bartered for human qualities here. Is that true?
John:	Of course it's true.
Mary:	I want some freedom. I want a whole lot of it. Do you have it here?
John:	Of course I have it! But you'd better watch your tongue, I don't deal with doubters. What kind do you want?
Mary:	I don't want to be so confined when I walk around the forest. I want to be free to go all over. I don't want to have to worry about the men with guns or the cars on the road. I want to be free.
John:	What are you willing to give me in exchange? I have three fine cups of freedom, just the kind you want. What have you got?
Mary:	I don't know . . . I'm just a young fawn. Do you know anything I have you want? What do you want? (*She is hesitant and somewhat embarrassed.*)

Like many magic shop customers, Mary has a hard time answering the shopkeeper's questions. The director can provide help:

Director:	Let's have some coaching from the audience, O.K.? Are there any other forest creatures here that want to kibbitz and make suggestions? (*Providing an example*) I'm a hawk and I say don't let that old lizard intimidate you, little fawn.
Group member:	I'm another old lizard and I know we lizards need a lot of what you've got. Why don't you offer him some of your youth and beauty?
Mary:	Oh no! I couldn't do that! That's me. I can't change who I am.
Group member:	I'm a bird. Don't give him anything. You're fine the way you are.

Mary: Oh, he would just go away. (*Shopkeeper nods vigorously.*) And it really wouldn't be fair. . . . Let's see . . . Oh, I know! I'll give you some of my ability to jump over fences and bushes, my agility. But not all of it, I need some for myself. I'll give you one cup.

John: I'll take it. I'm agile enough, but I am getting older. What else have you got? Let's go. I'm tired of waiting.

Mary: (*suddenly lights up with a sense of real understanding*) I know what I'll offer you. Something you really need. I'll offer you a cup of love. That's both loving and being loved. You really need that. And I've got a lot of it. Think how your life would change.

John: (*reacting with some surprise and smiling a rare smile*) You got me . . . I really do need that. Few of my customers seem to have any to give. . . . A cup? . . . No, that's too little. I want all of it. Give me all of it and I'll give you all my freedom (*laughs*). I don't need any here in the tree, so I'm way ahead.

Mary: I can't do that. If I give you all my loving I'll just get old and crotchety like you. I don't want freedom that badly. What's the use of being free when you're all alone?

John: (*very cold*) Let's cut the sermon. All or nothing.

Mary: Wouldn't you compromise?

John: No. All for all.

At this point, the director may have to help the bargainers come to a conclusion. I often find it helpful to participate by role-playing an audience member:

Director: We other forest animals demand that you bring this bargain to an end. This has gone far enough! (*Other group members join in readily, relieved they can express their impatience.*)

Group member: I'm a squirrel and I say, "Nuts to you." Go to another shop.

Group member: Yeah, this guy isn't going to give you any bargain. Leave.

Mary: Well, it doesn't look like I'll get what I want. . . . I'll have to go. . . . But I'm really sad. . . . Are you sure?

John: Of course I am.

Mary: I don't like it. I'll have to keep my guard up. Be careful. Watch that I don't get hurt. But at least I'll get some loving. (*Leaves slowly.*)

Like many of life's choices, many magic shop bargaining sessions remain unresolved. For our purposes, resolution is of little importance. The metaphoric content and the process of bargaining provide a rich soil for self-exploration. The group's understanding of the metaphor depends on its tele, on the group members' ability to tune in to each others' meanings intuitively. John's gruffness was easily recognized as the quality that made it difficult for staff members and clients alike to get a word with him in his office. His own recognition of his lack of warmth was enthusiastically received by the group—if he could admit it, maybe he wasn't quite so bad. Mary's characterization of herself as a pretty, vulnerable, naive creature of the forest seemed accurate enough for those of us who knew her.

After a magic shop scene is concluded, I try to focus the group members' attention on the bargaining process by asking, "How did you feel the bargaining went? What kind of bargainers did you see?"

In our scene, John responded immediately. Looking around at the downcast and exasperated expressions of the faces of several group members, he said, somewhat sadly, "Well, that's what my wife says about me, too. All or nothing. I just can't compromise. She could sure see me as a cranky old lizard who lives all by himself."

Most of the group members who had sided with Mary were a little surprised when she also expressed sadness about the bargaining. "This is the way it always happens. I talk and talk and then nothing changes. I don't know why I always seem to choose guys like that old lizard to bargain with."

In the next stage of the psychodrama we look at possible future work. I may ask the bargainers, "Now what do you want to do? Mary, do you want to explore another way of bargaining with a double?" Or we may want to work with John. "John, how about choosing someone to play the role of your wife and going home to tell her about today's magic shop?"

John was eager to work. Mary was not. John enacted a scene with his wife exploring the "all-or-nothing" bind using a double. John's stubborn loneliness touched off several other magic shops where the barter centered on love. When the magic shop develops into a successful bargain—a mouse, for example, is able to trade some of her ability to look helpless for an ounce of self-confidence—it can be developed by asking, "What are you going to do differently now? Now that you have that ounce of poise, whom do you want to meet?"

The role of the shopkeeper can be played with at least two radically different strategies. The first strategy, more often picked by inexperienced players, was demonstrated by our cranky lizard. The shopkeeper bargains for what he himself wants and needs. Both shopkeeper and shopper learn something about the ways in which each wants to change and what the costs of such change might be. With the second strategy, the shopkeeper uses his position to bring the shopper to a deeper level of exchange, by guessing what she would truly have to give up in order to gain what she wants.

He: I'm a beautiful golden statue of the Buddha.

She: I know, and I'm a butterfly. I'm just as beautiful as you are and I want strength.

He: What kind of strength?

She: Strength to oppose the wind and to wrench open the mouths of chameleons that want to eat me so I can escape.

He: I'll give you some strength but you won't always know when it comes.

She: What do you mean?

He: Sometimes you'll be able to oppose the wind alright, but sometimes you'll just want to brush someone with your lovely wings and it will hurt them.

The butterfly has to risk giving up the security of her own harmlessness. A snail who wants the lion's power must risk destroying his own shell. A hummingbird who desires peacefulness may need to know that she will have to give up some of her ability to move at an instant's notice. The mole who wants to bargain for sociability and friendship may have to give up some of his ability to dig himself into a deep private hole.

This kind of shopkeeper makes it clear that—all too often—the shopper does not want to (in contrast to: isn't able to, cannot, doesn't have a chance to) obtain the quality he seeks because it means giving up something crucial in return.

One of my favorite fairy tales in early childhood was the tale of the princess who couldn't stop crying. With the help of a witch who lived at the end of an arduous trail in one of the princess's forests, she traded her tears in for a magical necklace of laughter. The bargain was a poor one—because the princess had wanted to laugh instead of cry. Now, every time she found herself in a situation that would once have moved her to tears, she laughed, laughed as uncontrollably as she had cried before, and the necklace of beads danced and jingled along. Needless to say, she spent another long period of her life retracing that same arduous trail through the forest until she found the witch and returned the fatal necklace. Our magic shopkeepers often encounter princesses with equally foolish wishes. We hope, through the bargaining, to increase their wisdom. Some examples follow.

Burt is a longstanding member of one of our couples' groups. He is a mild-mannered, gentle, youngish man who speaks in a soft, appealing voice. The group is familiar with the underside of his smooth exterior. Burt is our champion procrastinator. He is as stubborn as a mule. He charms the others into helping him. But he will not move. Any suggestion is seen as a demand. He won't respond to demands. And he doesn't know what he could do on his own. So he doesn't move. He has come to my magic shop asking to buy the ability to work. He has no job. His wife is tired of supporting the family and he feels she has a point. But he can't get himself to do anything. He can't do the little jobs that need doing around the house; he can't seem to work on his art projects; he can't think what job he might seek. But he comes to my magic shop. He sighs. As shopkeeper, I ask him what he's offering in exchange for the quality he wants. I know already what I want and I'm waiting for the right moment to pounce.

He offers me pride. I take some, saying he'll need some for later and I add wryly that I'm not too interested in pride, especially in the absence of real achievements. Burt and I know each other well enough to allow bantering. He offers me a little of his creativity. The other group members counsel him against giving me any of it. I say I don't have that much demand for creativity without joy, anyway. I take a pound, again without much enthusiasm. I'm a very snooty shopkeeper. He offers me enthusiastic self-confidence, the feeling, when he starts, that whatever he's doing is going to be terrific, the best of its kind. I accept. But it's like his pride; I know it won't last and am reluctant to take too much. He still hasn't come up with what I want. I take two cups of confidence. He can't think what I want. He doesn't have anything else to offer. He looks wan. Full of self-pity. Status quo.

I begin to pounce. "How about your freedom of choice? Your freedom to do whatever you want all day long?" He reacts with a mixture of surprise and anger. Then he smiles, "Wow, my first reaction was you can't have any of that!"

I pounce again. "I want all of it. Well, almost all—ninety-nine percent of what you have." The bargain is on. Now he is really involved. He can't understand that any human being should be asked to give up freedom of any kind. I let him know that I need a lot of it since a lot of people will barter some of their most valuable properties for very small amounts. I also let him know that I think he will still have plenty of choice about his daily schedule even if he gives me ninety-nine percent of what he has. He will still have more than most people he knows.

He asks a lot of questions. He offers nothing. There is no bargain.

After a week has passed, Burt comes back to my magic shop. He has changed his mind. His freedom isn't doing him all that much good anyway. He just broods and aches with it. He'll take the bargain. The other group members see that Burt has taken the initiative. For the first time he seems to be taking a serious look at his own behavior. They take advantage of the chance to talk to Burt about his problems; for once, he doesn't seem put off by them. He feels ready to end his procrastination. My co-therapist suggests testing Burt's resolution by actually letting some of the group members check on his activities. Burt likes the idea. He is to receive a phone call at the end of each day for the next week, during which he is to account for his day's work. The following week, Burt appears more energized and reports that he has found a job. For the time being, he has worked himself out of his impasse.

Barbara, a young woman in her early twenties who is a member of an individuals' group at our center, came to my shop wanting the ability to handle her class of fifth graders more successfully. We had already spent some time role playing her class, and, as fifth graders, immediately found our teacher's weak spot. *She took every-thing personally. We were just kids doing whatever we could to amuse ourselves in a boring situation. And it was easy to amuse ourselves because she got uptight at the slightest provocation. Her face got all tense. She threatened punishments she didn't carry through. Mostly, it was her voice, though. She whined. What a drag.*

In my magic shop, Barbara offered her intelligence, her discipline, her depression, her creativity, as I bided my time for the pounce. This time I said: "Will you give up the hope that the kids in your class will make you feel that you are a good person?"

Again, the instantaneous reaction. Barbara clutched her stomach and said, "My first thought is, no, you just can't take that away from me." We bargained awhile. I let her know—zen-master fashion—that only in giving it up might she gain what she wanted; that being a good person might be the subject for another magic shop.

Barbara did not make a bargain. She is still thinking about it.

A magic shop bargain can be amazingly effective. In one instance, a young man who had been subsisting on welfare payments because of his inability to find work chose to go to a magic shop run by an ancient Tibetan Lama who lived high up in the mountains in a city carved out of rock by his loyal followers. In order to get there, he disguised himself as a mountain goat—skittish, lacking in patience, but strong and lithe enough to scale the most difficult of mountain terrains.

Lama: What do you want?
Goat: I want to be able to hold a job. I want some confidence and some patience so I can stay put instead of jumping and bolting at the slightest perturbance.
Lama: What do you offer me in return?
Goat: I don't have much. I could offer you some skittishness. Somebody who had trouble smelling danger could use it, maybe. I have no trouble with that at all.
Lama: Sadly enough, I have a lot of that quality already. Many of my customers lately seem to have an oversupply. But I could use a cupful. It would hardly make a dent in your stock, I'm afraid.
Goat: I want a really large supply of confidence to last out all those situations where I get scared. I need an ocean

of confidence and all I've offered you is a cupful of
skittishness. Could you use my ability to survive on very
little? I've been living on welfare for more than a year
now.

Lama: I could use that. In this materialistic age, it's a sought-
after quality. Will you give me all of yours?

Goat: No, I still might need it sometime. I'll give you seventy-
five percent, how's that?

Lama: I'll take it.

Goat: Is it enough?

Lama: No.

Goat: Do you see anything else you want?

Lama: I want your helplessness. It's a very effective variety.
You've been able to get others to give you food, money,
therapy. A lot of my customers need that variety of
helplessness. And you won't need it anymore if you have
confidence and patience, so give me all of it.

Goat: All of it? Then I'll never be able to get any help if I
need it. No. I'll give you seventy-five percent again, is
that enough?

Lama: It's a bargain, if you want it. An ocean of confidence
and patience for a cupful of skittishness and seventy-
five percent of both your ability to survive on very little
and your ability to be effectively helpless.

Goat: I'm afraid it'll be pretty scary sometimes, but I accept.

The bargain worked. The young man took his confidence job-
hunting with him, landed a job, and kept it for the entire following
year. In fact, he may still have it, as the writer has heard nothing to
the contrary.

Some of the best magic shop bargains end without resolution.
But even when that is so, the magic shop often serves to clarify an
impasse. The shopper may need to return to his impasse again and
again before he can see his way clear to resolving it. Meanwhile, the
bargaining continues.

Magic shop is a special technique: playful, sensitive, poetic. And
it has all the disadvantages of other such animals. Mood and atmosphere have to be right. The group has to be verbal and willing
to play. The more imaginative the group—college kids, teachers,

therapists, artists, children—the more likely the success. When the group aura is one of sound scientific reasoning, cautious self-reflection or other exclusively hard-nosed approaches, it will be difficult to run a magic shop. Some group members may have to get over a feeling of being condescended to or infantilized by the director; others may become bored with the somewhat abstract nature of the bargaining. The magic shop is a powerful technique, but limited. The time must be right. It can't be repeated very often.

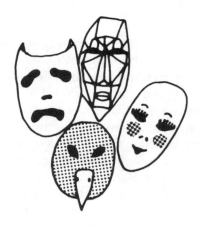

11

Masks

Bari Rolfe, a modern dancer who developed the art of mime together with the use of masks as a tool for drama students inspired my own use of masks with psychodrama. The mime's primary organ of emotional expression is her body. Her body "speaks" because her face is painted a stark white and her body covered in black. She keeps her face still. If one wants to eliminate facial gesture altogether in order to enhance the expression of the body, the face can be covered by one unvarying expression: the expression of the mask.

Masks are easy to construct. Simple instructions can be found in any book on the use of paper-maché. Halloween masks, pie tins, and the fiberglass forms found in equipment packages serve easily as molds. Books on theater arts give instruction in the use of lighter, plastic materials for making masks by taking impressions of actual faces, store room dummy faces, or other masks. In one group, we spent two delightful Saturday afternoons making masks—an activity which in itself spurs the imagination and helps build group cohesion.

Masks can represent any of the basic human qualities. They are particularly useful for exploring the polarities of human expression:

youth-age; seriousness-foolishness; beauty-ugliness; meanness-kindness; coldness-warmth. Bari works with one additional mask: the universal mask, a mask designed to suggest common humanity. The universal mask is neutral in skin tone; the features are classical and somewhat bland. Its nearest relative is the face of an unmade-up storeroom dummy; it suggests neither comedy nor tragedy. Even more than the expressionless face of the mime, this mask gains meaning only through movement.

When Bari began a series of classes for a group of therapists interested in developing the mask as an experiential tool, I joined. I found that she worked very much the way I had in my first psychodrama group. She gave us the same exercises she used with her actors and dancers, hoping that we would find our own application. I found that all of these exercises can be used as a warm-up and developed for further enactments.

We began simply. A trunk full of fifteen or twenty masks was brought to our group room, from which all the furniture had been removed. Instead of the usual assortment of pillows and lamps, the room was bare save for a full-length mirror brought in especially for the exercises. Bari suggested that we examine the masks and choose one that appealed to us, any mask that struck an emotional chord. We were then encouraged to try on the mask, work with it in front of the mirror, move our heads and upper bodies in ways that seemed to suit the mask, and, finally, to find the mask's walk.

The masks looked small and unassuming at first sight. They were a grayish white or skin color. Their expressions were extreme and often grotesque. I thought, as I put mine on, that it would never fit my face; it seemed out of proportion, the wrong color. As I moved it around, adjusting it to my face and hair, I soon changed my mind. It quickly became part of me. And, as I looked at the others in the room, half-expecting an embarrassing version of Halloween, I saw that they, too, were fitting into their masks.

We began to experiment with new body positions and movements to fit our masks. All of the therapists in the room knew each other well, yet when I looked around, the others had become strangers. When I looked in the mirror, I found myself unrecognizable as well.

I had chosen the mask of an old, wrinkled person with a discouraged and at the same time forbearing expression. The mask was much larger than my own face. As I began to arrange my hair around it in an effort to make it look more natural, I found myself feeling heavier and sadder. My head drooped further forward. My back rounded. My elbows locked at my sides, leaving only my forearms and hands to make futile, small gestures. I walked slowly. When I encountered other maskers I felt like the eternal grandmother: touching people lightly, making clucking noises that seemed both old and very young, shaking my head in what seemed both an affirmation of the other person and a resignation to my own burdensome existence. The mood was not familiar. I usually move quickly, stopping only for a reason. My usual stance is energetic, not resigned; yet putting on the mask had created the mood perfectly. I had become a composite of many of the old women I had known.

We didn't quite recognize each other. Over and over again, we had the experience of looking at someone we knew well and having to take a moment to remember who it was we were seeing. The mask simplified our perception of the others like a videotape with the sound turned off. And in addition to being deprived of the familiar voice we were deprived of facial expression. Just as many of us find out over and over again that we rely on words and thoughts and therefore fail to comprehend much of the emotional output which is coming our way, many of us became aware of being face-watchers during this exercise. What a shock to be confronted with an unmoving face! Some of us missed the subtlety of the others' expressions so much that we began to believe that the masks were changing— raising an eyebrow, pulling down a corner of the mouth, etc.! We had become so hungry for facial expression that we were reading into the mask what we saw in the expression of the body.

There are at least three advantages to the use of this very simple exercise. First, the mask, like the magic shop, gives permission to the wearer to experiment with surplus reality. Second, the wearer finds himself disguised in a way that affords him new insight into the way his body moves. Displayed against the unfamiliar mask, her body movement stands on its own. Third, the wearer of the mask experiences a marked change in the reactions of others to him. We often forget that we are as accustomed to the responses we elicit as to those we give. We're not only used to acting a certain way, but we rely on others to react to us in a certain way as well. The mask enables the wearer to experience herself in a new context.

Throughout Europe, where I grew up, there are traditional celebrations where masks are worn. The Bavarian *Fasching* lasts for several
days; the masked ball only an evening; the Tyrolean peasants' *Walpur-
gisnacht,* one whole night. European folklore is filled with tales of
the adventure, trickery, and supernatural events that happen on
these nights. These emotionally charged celebrations have an obvious appeal to the psychodramatist.

The mask taught me that the masquerader can, for a brief period,
step into another life in an entirely new way. She has to move, sense,
and see differently. She can experiment with being another person
far removed from her everyday self. Perhaps most important, others
will respond to her differently. No other form of self-disguise is so
successful. Masked, she will experience not being recognized by
those who know her. She will experience others reacting to a different
person inside her own skin.

In the next exercise, we used the universal mask. The object was
to make our movements congruent with its universality; in short, to
portray Everyman.

EXERCISE FOR USE OF UNIVERSAL MASK

Directions: "I want you to play the role of a human being who existed
much earlier in time, in much more primitive conditions. You will
be alone. You have spent a night sleeping in the forest. This is the
time when you awaken. Remember that what we want to see is what
might be the most basic characteristic of any human being in this
situation. We don't want to see particularities such as whether the
person is happy or unhappy, how old she is, whether she has a
headache. Just give us the basics. What does she experience, see,
touch? How does she move? It will help you if you focus on your
surroundings. React to them in the most simple, economical way
you can.

The immediate effect of the neutral mask is to blank out the face
and enhance the body. As I looked at myself wearing the regular-
featured mask, I found myself becoming even more aware of my
body movement than with the other masks. Because the face revealed
nothing in particular, I was able to look at the way I moved with the
kind of objectivity usually reserved for viewing others. Looking in

the mirror, I thought: *My shoulders tend to draw up. What an erect position! Isn't that a little stiff? Try to relax, Eva. Why carry one hand in front of your body as though you're carrying a purse? There is no reason why you can't just let your arms drop to your sides. Don't walk so hesitantly. Just walk.* Gradually, I eliminated some of the peculiarities of my way of moving.

As the exercise continued there was a sense of achievement and pleasure. I had chosen a relaxed, quiet walk to fit the mask. The exercise of awakening in the forest on a warm summer day delighted me. The experience of projecting something basically human translated to a new awareness of "belonging."

As we continued to work with all of the masks, the exercises became more and more complex. We each explored the use of different masks—different selves—working out short improvisations suggested by the masks. We worked individually, with one or two partners, or as a group. The usual acting exercises for group improvisations work equally well with masks. After everyone in the group has selected a mask, the group is told, for example, that they will spend the next twenty minutes portraying people caught in an air-raid shelter during World War II, or in the waiting room of a doctor's office, or at a once-a-year bargain-basement sale in a large city. There is, of course, one very important difference between the masked improvisations and other acting exercises: the mask demands silence. All communication has to be mimed.

I would not use the masks with a low functioning group because the mask can be threatening. Its visual effect alone can be bewildering.

MASK EXERCISES IN COUPLES GROUP

Another of the exercises with masks may be used with married couples. The couple is instructed to find character masks that illustrate an aspect of the relationship. I vividly recall my experience in doing this exercise with my husband.

As we stepped up to the trunkful of masks, I already knew the mask I'd choose. It was a mask I'd worn for years as a teenager and young woman, a little mask that had taken a great deal of hard work to shake off, that still returned in times of stress. Its most prominent feature was a grin, a very large grin that tyrannized every other feature of the face, spreading from ear to ear. The forehead was wrinkled, there were deep furrows at the sides of the mouth, and the small round eyes were barely visible beneath the folds of the all-encompassing smile.

Alan, meanwhile, had also chosen a mask. It was the opposite of mine. Where mine was small, his was large; mine was wrinkled, his smooth. While mine could have been either a woman's or a man's face, his was decidedly masculine. When I first looked at him with the mask on, he looked like the classic villain. The mask's smooth, large face was highlighted by prominent cheekbones and small, slitty eyes. The mouth was thin and, to my view, menacing. The most striking aspect of the mask was its blankness—it was smooth and cold.

We were to relate to each other for a few minutes and portray the part of ourselves which the masks represented. I began to "make nice." I wanted to be cheerful, to help out, to put a good face on things (a fitting metaphor), to help Alan and myself stay in a sort of pleasant limbo which would keep any strong emotion from being felt.

As I flitted about, touching Alan here and there, bringing him some food, chucking him under the chin, miming my little cheerfulness, I found, to my surprise, that he was portraying a character who was not in the least menacing. In fact, as he continued, I realized that menace would have been a relief in comparison to the character he was portraying. He was playing a passive, docile, and helpless person. The more I flitted, the more he sagged. He seemed not to know what to do about anything. He required help every step of the way. After our snack, I wanted him to help me with the dishes. Slowly he got the idea. Then he started dropping dishes. He didn't know where to put them when he had dried them. And he looked more and more sad and helpless. He never laughed at my jokes.

Little did I know with what vehemence I could be thrust back into my old cheery rescuer role. The more helpless Alan looked, the more frantic I felt inside. I had to cheer him up. I couldn't leave him to his own devices. I couldn't for a moment let either of us see who he was without help or who I was without helping. I rushed about, compulsively taking charge of both our actions and glossing over his failures when they occurred.

The members of our group (all of whom knew each other and the two of us quite well) responded to our scene with laughter. The extremes of our positions were familiar and the miming presented them in a comic form. For Alan and me, the exercise still serves as a reminder of one of the ways we get into trouble.

The directions I use for the couples' exercise with masks are as follows: "I would like each of you to choose a mask which has meaning for you in terms of your relationship to your husband or wife. This is a nonverbal exercise and I want you to choose the mask without talking. When each of you has put on your mask, I want you to mime a regular household activity together. It doesn't matter who starts; the other will get the idea of what you're doing and will join you. Remember the mask you are wearing and behave the way the mask directs you to behave. We will have four or five minutes for this exercise."

The couples' exercise can be used both in a group and during a regular clinical hour. One can elaborate the exercise in several ways, using both mirror and video-feedback to help people see themselves. (1) We ask members of each couple to choose masks for each other, and then perform the same exercise. (2) Each couple is asked to choose masks representing different aspects of their relationship: harmony, disharmony, the relationship at an earlier time, in the future, etc.

In our couples group, we found the technique to be particularly fruitful in testing projections. The husband who put a bitter mask on his wife, for example, found, as she began to play her scene with him, that he no longer experienced her in this way, that the bitterness of her mask was familiar, but more as a memory of the past. Another couple surprised the group when the wife selected as an ideal a mask that would have been perfect for a football player as the mask she would like to see her husband wear. She had spent much of the group's time complaining about his lack of feeling. Now she seemed to be saying that it was she who preferred the strong, silent type.

Each exercise can be developed further. For example, when there is a strong response to a particular scene in the couples group, we often ask other couples to do the same exercises using the masks the others wore. This enables us to look at typical marital conflicts: introvert-extrovert, witch-victim, villain-victim, victim-rescuer, stone-face-hysteric, etc. Any exercise can be intensified by asking the players to redo a scene by pushing it to an extreme:

Directions: "If this mask represented your life for the next ten years, how do you two think you'd be relating to each other then? Let's see you ten years later.

Before you start, give yourself a few minutes to take stock of your present state of mind. How do you feel now, at the end of this scene? What feels familiar? What feels strange? What is your mood like? What do you feel toward your partner? What is your body telling you? Are you feeling tense or relaxed? If you are tense, where is the tension located? If you exaggerated that tension more and more, what would happen to your body? Close your eyes, if you wish, and let yourself answer these questions. Think and feel what might happen to you after ten more years of this kind of existence. In a few minutes, we'll take a look at you two as you would be in ten years." Quick responses must be discouraged in this exercise. It depends on the participants' taking enough time to explore their experiences.

This method of intensification is applicable to many of the techniques described in this book. An individual who has arranged a sociogram can be asked to relate to those same individuals after ten years, for example. A group doing a drawing together for a warm-up exercise can be asked to take stock of themselves and fantasize where ten years of a similar process would lead them.

Masks can also be used to work with families of origin. In a technique developed by Justine Fixel, MSW, the protagonist is asked to find masks for her parents and herself. The masks—as many and varied as possible—are displayed on a table so that she can make her choice. She then chooses members of the group to take the roles, which must be mimed. The directions are to find a scene which symbolizes the relationship. The scenes are usually short and powerful. Devil fathers toying with angel mothers; both parents in golden masks revolving around a mirror. Often, the mask evokes ancient ritual. There is a sense of sacred space. The director's job is different here: she must allow the scene to be observed rather than develop it further. The staging of this scene will be remembered for a long time.

Using these exercises with various groups of clients, I have come to think that they are of particular value to groups composed of individuals with a high degree of verbal skills. They have the advantages of other nonverbal exercises in breaking through the verbal, intellectualizing defenses and, they provide an unusually potent catalyst for the use of the imagination. For individuals who are flexible and confident enough not to be threatened by the sheer outrageousness of a room full of people disguised by grotesque masks, these group exercises are energizing. At times, they even lead to that process so little known in the hallowed halls of group therapy: having fun.

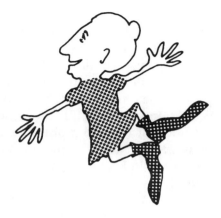

12

Permission for Spontaneity

Clinicians are accustomed to hearing bad news. Our clients come to us with tales of woe about the past and tales of sorrow about the present. We are called upon to listen, to help our clients make sense of what is happening to them and support them. We sometimes forget that we can play another role, one that is healing without being nearly so depressing. We can provide a new context for our clients, a larger context that enables both client and therapist to experiment with different roles, and in the process, develop a more flexible, spontaneous relationship.

If we let our office walls listen only to the sadness of the past and the hopelessness of the present, we may soon be depleted of whatever small amount of healing power has been given us. If, on the other hand, four office walls can be changed at will to a carnival, to another planet, to a submarine, there's hope that something different can occur both for ourselves and for our clients.

Both clinician and client inhabit a culture where a sort of dreary sense of responsibility is paraded constantly while spontaneity is feared and suppressed. At worst, the clinician often finds himself rigidly bound by the role of a therapist: a quietly dressed, softspoken, kindly but slightly impersonal individual who carefully avoids using vivid language and limits himself to short questions and short answers. All too frequently, his client is equally bound. He knows that he is to come in and talk about problems. He cultivates a downcast expression, a thoughtful brow, often speaks even more softly than his therapist (the therapist appears to be suggesting that speaking up is wrong), and cannot imagine saying that anything good is happening in his life or engaging the therapist by telling a joke, for example. (Well, perhaps he can imagine it, but he knows better than to try it.) Both therapist and client have fantasies, intuitions, and associations during the hour which are well within their awareness but which they label inappropriate to the lofty work in which they are engaged. Needless to say, these are stereotypes, but they exist not only in individual therapy; they exist in groups, in families, in all but a few select spots of our cultural environment.

Let us assume that the clinician knows the boundaries of the relationship. She knows that there are rules about inappropriate behavior which should never be violated. Spontaneity and impulsivity are not the same. Spontaneity, as Zerka Moreno stresses, is an appropriate reaction to a new situation, not a license to act out.

Within these boundaries, the psychodramatist is the enemy of the constricting stereotype. She's an iconoclast. She frequently does the unexpected and asks his clients to do the same. She gives permission to be spontaneous, to experiment, to try out something ludicrous, something potentially embarrassing, something new. We have talked about the clinical use of techniques such as doubling, role reversal, magic shop, and the use of masks, but we have not talked enough about the powerful meta-message given by the purveyor of these techniques.

A therapist who starts talking about a shop that deals in human qualities, who owns a trunkful of masks, who suddenly gets up and talks for another person, is modeling spontaneity. She is giving permission to play. She is giving permission to talk and listen at several levels: the level of content and information, the level of drama, the level of fantasy, and the level of play. By participating in some of the scenes she sets up, she is modeling a way out of the tales of woe, a way to take an active part that may prove to be enjoyable, exciting, even anxiety-provoking. She is giving permission to experiment, to play, and to change.

We often think of therapy as reparenting. The therapist who can play is clearly one of the most enjoyable substitute parents. She will encourage her child to grow, to dare to be different, and she will be able to model both the excitement of play and the serious intensity of a therapeutic relationship.

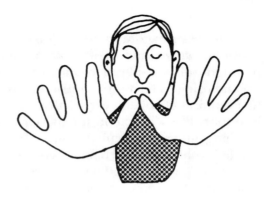

13

Resistances and Some Ways of Dealing with Them

The basic resistance is always the same: fear of change. We want to become different but we dread it. Whether we are confronting helpful friends or relatives, a priest, a therapist, or a group, there's always a part of each of us that wants to experiment, to risk, to venture forth into the unknown, and part that holds back—conservative, frightened, paranoid—quick to judge the risk foolish, ridiculous, wrong. Much has been written about resistance to various forms of psychotherapy. Here we will concentrate on resistance to psychodrama and how we can help them overcome it.

The first level of resistance to psychodrama is stagefright. We all associate dramatic work with performing for others, being looked at, being found out. *I can't go on stage. Everyone will notice what I'm really like. They'll find out how dumb (awkward, silly, fat, unworthy, ugly, crazy) I really am. I won't be able to hide. I'd be too ashamed. This is an exercise in humiliation.* Participating in a psychodrama means exposing a vulnerable self to others who may not understand.

Both the protagonist and the auxiliary risk exposure while entering unknown territory. They fear losing the familiar sense of self by playing a role outside the boundary of their accustomed behavior. Volunteering to be a protagonist means showing a part of one's life that requires change. It carries the risks of washing one's dirty linen in public. Every protagonist experiences, to some degree, the fear of being judged, ridiculed, found "lacking in the basic qualities needed to be a human being," as one of my students put it. To be oneself on stage is paradoxical. One is oneself in one's most private moments. How can one portray the self? How can one behave naturally on a stage?

For the auxiliary, fitting into the role of another also carries risks. Idiosyncrasies such as tone of voice, quality of language, gestures, and rhythm of movement help each of us identify ourselves. At times of stress we cling with desperation to our identifying characteristics. The thought of acting the role of another person may have great appeal—it offers a rich soil for trying out aspects of ourselves we've neglected—yet we resist, afraid that somehow the old self won't be the same thereafter, afraid of the unknown self which may emerge.

The question "Who am I" looms large on our culture's alienated horizon; role playing often appears as a threat. *Does playing a role well mean that a part of my true self is emerging? What if I like myself better the way I usually am? One way to handle it is just to play nice people. That way I won't take a chance. Another way is not to take part at all—"I'm just watching."*

When in doubt, say, "I can't." It's a nice way of saying "I won't," it lets both of us off the hook. If I can't do it—well, that means I would if I could. And you obviously can't ask me to do something I'm unable to do.

The "I can't" is a familiar maneuver in any resistance game. In psychodrama, the "I can't" often means, "I can't act." The individual knows that "he can't do it." He is not skilled enough, not smart enough, not brazen enough. He is embarrassed. He appears to have stage fright. *I can't act; I can only be myself. . . . I couldn't do that in front of all these people. . . . I don't know how she's feeling, how could I act like her? . . . I never even met his mother, I can't be like her. I'm too embarrassed to try.*

An individual who feels threatened by the opportunity to role play may resist by questioning its basis or attacking it as a harmful activity. *Role playing is a game which will only teach me to play more artificial games. Role playing is dangerous because it will distort my view of reality and drive me crazy.*

Both types of resistance present serious problems to the psychodrama director because, as all of us who have led other types of groups know, resistance is highly infectious. *If he can't do it; I can't do it. If he says it's bad for us, maybe it is bad for us.* It is important to consider these objections and arrive at some ways of handling them.

The warm-up is the most valuable antidote to resistance. No amount of explanation can supplant the simple messages given by a successful warm-up: this is a group where everyone can participate; participation is easy and fun; any contribution is rewarded. In structuring the warm-up, the director also gives the message that she is prepared to take responsibility for the functioning of the group. A group member learns that he will not be left to his own devices, struggling with his own fears because the warm-up can set up an atmosphere of spontaneity that eases the resistive trends in the group. At the end of the warm-up, most of the group members will have participated and the remainder will have learned that they won't be punished for resisting, only encouraged to participate.

Struggling with my own resistances and those of group members, especially the groups of people I see in acute states of crisis on hospital wards or in day centers, I have developed a style which is at some variance with "classical" or Moreno-style psychodrama. It consists largely of techniques which de-emphasize the aspect of "theater" or "staginess" in psychodrama and attempt to replace these with psychotherapeutic work that looks more like what goes on in other, more familiar therapy groups. The stage area can be anywhere in the room; it is usually either in the center of the circle around which we sit, or even part of it. There is no stage. If a person doesn't want to work in the middle of the room, I usually move the stage area to wherever he happens to be sitting and work from there. I may direct sitting next to him, to give him extra support. Neither is a "performance" required. If others can't hear the protagonist, I usually ask them to move nearer the area where she is working rather than asking her to speak louder. I don't want to ask the protagonist to feel that she has to produce her feelings in a louder voice than is comfortable and I have no objection to others sitting near her, on the floor, even if it doesn't quite fit the scene. I often discourage applause because I don't want to give group members the message that they have to be entertaining or entertained by what's going on. An empathic comment or a hug can be far more personal and supportive than the clapping of hands. Following an enactment in a small group, I ask those in the scene and those that watched to share what touched them about the enactment. The sharing period provides both an emotional outlet for the observers and an opportunity for the protagonists to hear strongly felt commentary.

Applause can also work as an energizer—when it breaks out spontaneously, at the point where a protagonist is achieving a moment of strength, for example, or when it is labeled as a way a large group can provide encouraging feedback and can be followed by individual comments.

These techniques counter the "I can't" resistance. All of them continue the message of the warm-up that anyone can participate, that there will be support from the director, and that no specialized skills are required. The director's own reaction to the "I can't" resistance is important. If she hears it as a statement of fact or a final evaluation of the person's abilities, she's at a loss. If she can hear it as information about a person's present state of mind in relation to trying a new and risky activity, she can begin to work. I usually assume that the person can do the work and doesn't know it. If a group member responds to a request to play a role by saying something like, "Oh, no! I couldn't do that. Pick somebody else," I usually respond in a very low-keyed manner intended to convey that I want to help her to give herself a chance to try. I may use any number of the following phrases: "Well, let's see, maybe you could give it a try, knowing that it's hard to start. You don't know yet whether or not you can do it . . . it just feels like it might be hard." I may also make suggestions that are intended to give the individual more control over her choice and counteract her feeling that she is making a fool of herself:

> *Director:*   (*to Joan*) How about trying to play John's wife and letting John decide how you're doing?
>
> *Director:*   (*to John*) John, if the way Joan plays your wife doesn't fit, will you stop the scene and let her know?
>
> *Director:*   (*to Joan, who looks reluctant*) Could you try it for a while and then stop to consider whether you want to con-

	tinue or get a replacement from the group?
Joan:	I don't think so. I don't think I can.
Director:	(*to Joan*) Are you saying "I can't" or "I won't"? If you really mean "I won't," then I won't say anymore; I don't want to pressure you. But try saying "I won't."
Joan:	What do you mean?
Director:	Say, "I won't" to me, to see if it fits for you.
Joan:	OK. Yeah, that's right. I won't do it. I don't want to do what you asked. I won't.
Director:	OK. You won't.

The last is a paradoxical intervention. On the one hand, the director is giving permission to rebel, to remain uncooperative. On the other hand, she asks for cooperation in repeating the words "I won't." This is an example of the creative double message developed by Milton Erikson, the medical hypnotist. It sets the stage for further cooperation.

Joan may want to say more about not wanting to participate or she may just want to sit back and watch. I will usually come back to her later to check whether different circumstances increase her desire to participate. In the event that Joan sticks to her original "I can't," I assume that she is telling me that she wants to try. I watch closely for any signs that indicate that Joan may be willing to change her mind. If I see her nodding her head, smiling, or making a move into the scene with John, I usually encourage her by remaining near her physically until she feels more comfortable. It very seldom happens that the individual uses the controls offered to her—to stop and ask for help, or stop and get a replacement. However, if she does, I make sure that her wish is respected. I assume group members attend because they want to participate. If the assumption proves false with a particular individual, I try to communicate two messages: that it's OK not to want to participate and that there'll be further opportunity to try in case he changes his mind. For example:

John:	I think this is ridiculous (*sounding very belligerent*). The other therapists here are trying to teach us to be more realistic and this is phony. It's artificial.
Eva:	That's true, it's artificial. It's a way of exploring by doing something artificial.

John:	Well, I'm not going to do it. It isn't going to help me, I don't think.
Eva:	That's OK. I'll probably come back to you every once in a while though, to see if you want to participate. Is that OK with you?
John:	(*nods head yes reluctantly*).

If John had not given his reluctant assent in the end, I would have accepted that response as well, asking him to stay around to see how the rest of it went. This strategy allows John to take a negative position without being punished for it, and saves the director from getting into a struggle with John which would probably prove to be useless as well as upsetting to the rest of the group members.

When, like John, the resisting individual questions role playing itself, some discussion may be in order. He may feel it's all phony or artificial or he may make a learned disputation on the impossibility of ever stepping into anyone else's shoes. His quarrel is not with his lack of ability to perform the task; he is stating his opposition to the very concept of psychodrama as a healing art. I have formulated my thoughts on these issues in the following monologue:

I am who I am. Psychodrama can't suddenly change that. I can't become someone else. I am who I am. I can, however, use various parts of myself to play different roles. Some of those parts may be close to what you already know about me. If I play Jane's girl friend, talking to her about why I think nobody else in the dormitory likes us, you may see very little difference from the Eva that leads psychodrama. A little softer maybe, a little chattier in her conversation. But pretty much the same Eva. If I play John's wife, accusing him of hurting my feelings, you will see an Eva that seldom appears in the psychodrama director, but you won't be terribly surprised. 'That's just the way she acts at home. She doesn't get that upset with us. Because we don't have that kind of power in her life,' you might think. You're right. I know the Eva I bring out when I play John's wife very well. My high-pitched, somewhat whiny voice. My tendency to say the same thing over and over. My injured air. But I don't usually trot this part of myself out in public.

Neither Jane's girl friend nor John's wife causes me much trouble. These— like many other roles in my daily repertoire—are roles which I know I play. I may not entirely approve of these parts of myself, but I recognize them; they are familiar, homey. The trouble starts when I use a part of myself I usually bury. I play Tamara, the well-known dance director. I am loud, manipulative, driving, manic. I move constantly. I have to have the others under my spell. I look deeply into each person's eyes. I can't rest. Can't stop. After the scene is over, you are amazed: 'That's really acting. That isn't like you at all.' I, on the other hand, feel slightly nauseated. That's a part of me alright. A part I don't show very often. A part I feel ashamed of. I feel a little shaky lest you now see me as 'that woman.' I need some time to be quiet and get back to being the Eva I know better. Then maybe I can make some sense of what happened. Another therapist helps me understand. I was playing a part of my mother I experienced as very painful. A person who frantically covers up her inner turmoil with activity, distraction, and power maneuvers. An isolated, lonely person, certain of her doom.

Of course, this is not a monologue to be delivered to the group. These are thoughts, memories, and reactions that underlie my work with resistant group members.

Role playing cannot be total make-believe. We can only act ourselves. But, because we are only aware of a limited part of ourselves at any given time, we often surprise ourselves. The surprise may be a delightful one. We discover a new richness of expression. The discouraged housewife acts the role of her teenage daughter with gusto. For a while, her depression seems to lift. She is no longer slow-moving, soft-voiced, and retiring in her gestures, but becomes mercurial in her emotions, loud, charming, repulsive—a typical teenager. A cantankerous young woman, feared by the other group members for her acid tongue, plays the role of a nurse who relates to an incoming client with a quiet softness and tenderness. The result is surprise *I didn't know I had it in me* and usually delight *I'm not just depressed, I'm not just sarcastic, and the others in the group can see this other part of me and like it.*

On the other hand, we may surprise ourselves in a way that leaves us feeling confused. After playing Tamara, a woman who had all kinds of qualities I despised, I experienced confusion, a feeling which says in essence: I don't know what just happened. *Playing the role felt very real to me. Yet I feel scared. I didn't know I could act like that. And now that I know, I don't think I can accept it. I don't like that part of me. I can't make any sense of it. I want to forget it. And I want the others to forget it. What if they think that's the real me?* Again, we are looking at the process of bringing into awareness an aspect of our behavior which is not a part of our daily repertory. Confusion, fear, and blocking often arise when we meet up with a part of ourselves we

don't understand or like. These feelings most often emerge with
negative roles: double-binding, sweetly hostile parents; provocative,
teasing wives; withdrawn, icy husbands.

Conflicts of this nature are potentially productive. If the director
counteracts the participant's tendency to disqualify the experience
with phrases such as: "That's not real, anyway. . . . I was only acting . . . in the real situation it would have been different," she can
help explore the conflict, and bring into awareness the person's
dilemma about showing a part of herself she usually hides. With
more understanding, the confusion lifts and the individual makes
gains: she may be able to reclaim a part of herself, she may discover
choices about expressing feelings hitherto suppressed. *I learn that I
can be strong, active, and vivacious without the desperate restlessness I sensed
in my mother. There is a part of me that's like my mother—I'm leading this
psychodrama, after all. I also know that I'm very different from her. I don't
have to be so careful. I can play the role of someone who resembles her without
becoming my mother.*

Members of therapy groups are often reluctant to play negative
roles: the mean mother-in-law, the nagging wife, the stern father.
We do not want to appear bad in front of others; even if we can
justify acting one of the villains as helping another person, we often
feel embarrassed to admit that we know how to play the villain's
game. One woman in our group had the classical Jewish mother.
Before she could play her in a scene with a Jewish man, she told us
she was afraid of acting the part—a whining, cajoling, cloying woman.
She was afraid playing her mother would be a cruel satire; to her
surprise, she learned a lot about her mother's passionate attachment
to her children from playing the role.

Sometimes negative roles are avoided because of the fear of losing
control. Asked to play an angry, punitive father, an individual fears
that he would become too angry and actually hit someone during
the roleplaying. A woman does not want to participate in a scene
involving grief for fear that she'll cry. If I detect these fears, I try to
make them explicit so that we can talk about what the next step
might be. We may decide that the scene can be stopped whenever
the individual feels it necessary. We may provide the son with a
pillow so that he can defend himself against Dad, if necessary. We
may give Dad a scene in which he does beat a pillow or mattress to
help him release some of his anger safely. The woman afraid of her

tears may need to do her own grief scene before she can participate in anyone else's. Or she may need to use a double that has the specific task of supporting and protecting her by asking questions that help her express what she needs to express at a comfortable pace. Or she may find out that she has less objection to crying in the group once she's talked about it.

One way in which groups give permission to act out negative roles is by modeling. In a new group, I often take on some of these roles myself at first and then, after I have started, ask whether anyone else in the audience is in touch with the person I am playing and could fill in for me. When someone in a new group does risk portraying negative roles or emotions, I make a point of reminding the group that she did us a favor by taking on this role, and comment that I hope group members realize that the portrayal was different from the way she usually presents herself. I also watch whether there is any hostile reaction from other members of the group, so that I can bring it out into the open. If hostility remains unexpressed, it will only add to the forces of resistance. After a short time—two or three meetings—a group usually develops an ethos more tolerant of villains. Playing the villain can be rewarding. Everyone knows that being good means giving up all the fun of being bad. In psychodrama groups, individuals can experiment with their bad potentialities without getting into trouble. In one of my groups, held in a day hospital where there were constant quarrels between the adolescent population and the adult population who shared the same recreation room, some of the most fruitful work came from a role reversal which allowed the adults to run about the stage, turning up the radio and jiving in time to the music, while their teenage counterparts became the moralizing martyrs. In a student group, one of the girls got insight into her own life when she role-played her mother and saw how manipulated the others felt by her. Many people spend their days playing a constricted, inhibited role that allows little expression of feeling, positive or negative. What better way to break out than to play someone's swearing, ranting, dissatisfied father?

Psychodrama directors often feel discouraged by group resistance. Our own resistances become stronger. We become severe judges of our own behavior and develop the same doubts and fears we face in our group members: *Should I really try to get them to do something they don't want to do? I don't now how to set up role playing all that well;*

can I blame them for saying they don't know how to do it yet? There is something phony about psychodrama. It would be easier just to talk. I've been trained to talk with people. I can do that. Let's just talk and forget the role playing for now. If someone is obviously having difficulty accepting a role he's played, or if he is clearly afraid of acting a role which may put him in a negative light, our resistance increases even more. *Do I have the right to ask him to take such a risk? What if it's really bad for him? What if he acts his angry father and he does lose control? Then what do I do? Furthermore, some kinds of strong feelings upset me, too. I don't want him to see me upset. I don't think I want him to take the risk. . . .*

For me, the greatest help has been to know that I can go slowly. I don't have to get the whole group involved in a psychodrama of great intensity in a matter of minutes. I can make suggestions and encounter the resistances step by step. I can follow. I give people choices about whether they want to work or not. There are some people for whom psychodrama does not fit. They've been conscious of doing so much acting all their lives that, paradoxically, the very thought of using it to gain self-awareness frightens them. I see myself as giving such individuals as clear a picture as possible of what the next step might be, but I know that I am not responsible for their taking it. If I see my role as supporting group members in making clear, responsible choices, I don't have to view each encounter as a struggle in which I'm on one side and the resisting person is on the other. I observe that the resisting person is in conflict: he is here and that says something about his desire to participate, but he's refusing to do so. I know that I can give him support for any clear choice. If he chooses "I won't" for a particular role or for the entire group, I can support that. If he chooses to take the next step, I'll support him there.

There is no right way to handle resistance. These examples are given as a basis for developing ways of handling the problems that come up in groups. Personal style is relevant to each and every technique we discuss; it is crucial in handling the delicate, subtle, important issues of resistances. We all know that children work out many of their questions about trust by testing limits; the same process takes place between group members and their directors. Consider the issues raised in this chapter and experiment with ways of handling them until you feel comfortable. The cohesiveness and trust in the group will depend on your solutions.

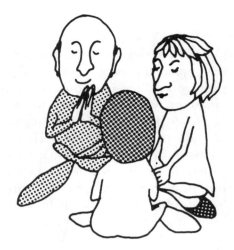

14

Trance and Psychodrama

Largely through the influence of Milton Erickson and his followers, a great deal of work on hypnosis and trance took place in the 'eighties. Its affinity with psychodrama first occurred to me when I was doing some personal work with Erickson and while in trance overheard him talking with my husband, who was also present. "You see," I heard him say, "she has achieved a really nice degree of relaxation. Her eyes have rolled back slightly. She is flushed. Her breathing has slowed down." I wasn't at all convinced that he was describing me accurately, but for some reason I didn't feel like making objections. Erickson seemed to believe I was in a trance state. I would not be so rude as to contradict him. Looking back on the experience, I know that I was, in fact, in a trance, a trance light enough to allow extraneous thoughts and deep enough to let me enter a world of memories that I hadn't known existed. Afterward, I learned that I had also experienced the physical manifestations of a trance. I yawned and stretched and felt a sensation of warmth and tingling in my arms. Something about the way Erickson talked had allowed me to have this experience without being fully aware of it.

It's not easy to describe the quality of Erickson's talk, because rather than simply explaining something to Alan, it seemed that he was "speaking for me," much like a psychodramatist who helps a protagonist by using doubling or soliloquy techniques. A more detailed analysis of Erickson's work revealed other similarities.

The hypnotist paces his subject; that is, he patterns the pace of his talk to the breath and rhythm of his subject's reactions. He analyzes his subject's primary way of perceiving the world—is it primarily visual, auditory, or tactile—and uses it to join the subject, only gradually leading her to a different experience through trance. The double also proceeds by working at the same pace and in the same mode as her protagonist. Both hypnotist and psychodramatist work toward a "joining" with the client. Neither indulges in repartee. The object for both is to become part of the protagonist's world, to help the protagonist change by infiltration rather than analysis, discussion, or role-modeling.

One way to discuss the similarity of trance and psychodrama is to return to the subject of critical distance last discussed in the chapter on doubling. The reader will recall that the term refers to the accepted norm of physical distance between animals, such as the distance between birds who land on the telephone wires or the distance beyond which a cat will attack another cat. These distances are regulated with mathematical accuracy in human beings as well. As people face each other across tables, across work places, as they discuss something while they walk together, sit together on a couch, or lie in bed together, they depend on the distance between them remaining fairly constant. Any change in distance usually signals a change of behavior and relationship. Distance regulates the ability to touch. Words like, "sir, madam, Mr., Mrs., kid, pal, friend, honey, dear" help indicate the proper distance. Once found, the distance is kept unless a change occurs in the relationship, at which point the distance also changes. Frequently, such changes are marked by rituals such as marriage and puberty rites. Critical distance means "safe" distance. It means that the talkers can rely on each other to stay in their own space, without risking intrusion or abandonment.

During an enactment, there is no assurance that the critical distance will be kept. The double often touches the protagonist; the others in the drama may move in and out according to how close they feel; they may even pile pillows on the protagonist to demonstrate that the relationship is smothering her. As a result, the protago-nist has difficulty maintaining her normal defenses. She may feel vulnerable and confused outside the safe boundaries of her accus-tomed world. She may even find herself opening up to spontaneous, creative change.

The trance state also calls for a change in critical distance. The hypnotist often touches his subject's lifted or limp arm, for example, or leans in closely to observe his subject's rate of breathing or skin color. At the same time, he talks in a way that overlooks the subject's otherness. He does not expect a social response. "You don't even have to listen to my voice," Erickson would say, as though only he were in the room talking to himself. How, then, could the subject find her accustomed distance? Both psychodramatist and hypnotist discourage conventional interaction. While the work is going on, it seldom occurs to the subject to say anything about what is going on, and if it does—as it did in my own case, the need to say it may mysteriously disappear. Both hypnotist and psychodrama director also tend to discourage talk after the session, so that the work won't get buried in intellectualization. If there is no discussion, how can the subject remain in her usually defended position? Instead, disori-ented by these techniques, the subject relies on her guide, the hypno-tist or psychodramatist. I believe that in both cases the subject is often in a trance.

But there is more. The protagonist has entered a new situation where, guided by trustworthy helpers, she often discovers a surprising ability to think, imagine, and behave differently. Both protagonist and hypnotic subject relate to a new-old story that will stir the uncon-scious mind. In Ericksonian hypnosis, she follows the story the hypno-tist weaves, a story relevant to her life in critical ways, one that often reveals to her the absurdity of her standard responses and enables her to wake from his trance refreshed, with a new point of view. In psychodrama, the protagonist helps tell her own story, and yet, de-spite the fact that the characters and the plot are the same, finds herself continually surprised and challenged by it. She sees the old familiar situation there on the stage, but experiences it in the here and now and reacts spontaneously. The others in her enactment make her feel freer to be herself. She is less defended. The role players and doubles seem to be able to frustrate and support her at the same time. Frequently she finds herself doing or saying things she had never dared do or say.

Both trance and psychodrama are founded in paradox. The hypnotist who says, "You don't even have to listen to my voice" plans every word as a message to his subject's subconscious. The subject, free not to listen, listens to every word. The psychodramatist provides a cast of characters who frequently represent an exaggerated version of the difficulties and frustrations of the protagonist. But both the director and the cast of characters are there to help the protagonist. Both hypnotist and psychodramatist take full charge of the session. At the same time, both frequently give the protagonist the sensation of being fully in charge for the first time. In the paradox, spontaneity and creativity are born.

Both hypnotist and psychodramatist provide an experience that by definition is extraordinary and thus has some of the quality of ritual or heightened reality. Unlike group and individual psychotherapies that rely mostly on the exchange of verbal information, psychodrama and hypnosis encourage the subject to enter a different world, the world of the past, of the future, of heightened intensity. Both use the "story" to frame the subject's dilemma. The hypnotist tells a story that on the surface may seem irrelevant to the subject, who soon discovers that he is at the very center of it. I remember Erickson telling one story after another about people he knew who were in a rut. *In a rut? Could he be referring to us? No! And yet it must be admitted that my husband and I did find ourselves climbing out of a few "rutlike" situations when we got home.* The psychodramatist arranges a drama in which the protagonist is the author and the star. Not unlike shamanic rituals such as the medicine wheel or sand painting, psychodrama and hypnosis both place the subject in the center and provide means to explore her dilemma that are both unfamiliar and traditional.

Psychotherapists vary in their views about the amount of responsibility they place on the client. Some feel that the hour is the patient's responsibility and make only minimal verbal responses tailored to echo the client's words and only add the subtlest changes to lead the client a little further. In general, their behavior is designed to give the message "This is your life. This is your session. You're the only one that can take charge." Others take a more parental role, providing conversation, explanations, and advice to their clients.

Their message is "You've come to me with your problem. I have experience in this area. I will help you work this out." Both hypnotist and psychodramatist take full responsibility for the session (see Chapter 1). The relationship resembles that of the priest or shaman in that the subject is encouraged to feel that she has come to someone who will arrange circumstances to help her heal. The protagonist is not in charge; the director is.

It is probably no coincidence that both hypnosis and psychodrama can be used as occasional as well as regular therapies. While there are many groups who meet weekly or monthly, it is not uncommon for a subject to attend a hypnosis session or a short series of sessions once or twice in her life or to go once and then return for a follow-up several years later. The same is true of psychodrama. The "healing" that takes place can be a single event of momentous importance in the subject's life or it can take place over time. The subject will recall bits and pieces of her work as she returns to her daily routine and discover change has taken place without her being aware of it.

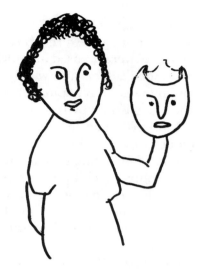

15

Psychodrama or Drama Therapy?

Both psychodrama and drama therapy use methods derived from the theater to enact and highlight human situations. Both disciplines are primarily known as group therapies, although practitioners of both have begun to work with individuals as well. How, then, are they different?

The most important difference, in my view, arises from the times of their birth; it is the difference between the early and the late 20th century. Psychodrama had its beginnings in Freudian Vienna while drama therapy developed primarily in England, Holland, Israel and the United States during the 1970's and 1980's. In the early part of the century, when psychotherapy itself was new and revolutionary, psychodrama was outrageously different from anything that had gone before. Even in the legitimate theater, improvisation, the basis of role-playing, was just beginning to cross the boundary of comedy and cabaret to the legitimate acting studio. By the time drama therapy came along, role-playing—a form of improvisation—had become widely accepted as a teaching technique in education, business, and psychotherapy, and improvisational theater had developed many new and exciting directions. Early in the century, nearly all the therapies were focused on individual healing. Later, group therapies developed and became widely adapted to many different therapeutic disciplines. This chapter will look at some of the ways psychodrama and drama therapy resemble each other, and how they differ.

Moreno began his career by using theater and story telling techniques to entertain children and do acts of social service. The accounts of his sitting under a tree at a playground, dramatizing stories for groups of children are as legendary as his volunteering, for example, to bring Vienna's prostitutes together with the police, using drama techniques to achieve better relations. When he came to the United States, he did so with the goal—with which he got quite far—of establishing a professional improvisational theater. Still, the critics were often unkind to this new form of theater and it was partly because of the frustration of New York's theater world, that Moreno, who was also a psychiatrist by training, developed his improvisational techniques to help people heal. Without the need to make money and impress critics, he felt he could make beautiful theater out of real human drama and help people to explore the truth and gain spontaneity—the keys to mental health. In my view, Moreno's trust in the protagonist's ability to heal himself through authentic, spontaneous interaction may be the only theory to come out of that very important period that focused on health, rather than pathology. Often confused with permission for impulsivity, Moreno, in fact stressed the learning of the appropriate spontaneous response, arguably the most important characteristic of the healthy personality.

Because his techniques were rooted in the theater, Moreno nearly always worked with groups, although the main focus of psychodrama is individual work. Psychodrama, though Moreno knew it helped audience and auxiliaries as well, was developed to help the protagonist, the center of every enactment. The others in the drama are auxiliaries: helpers. If one of the auxiliaries or a member of the audience is deeply affected by an enactment and there is time, that individual may become the protagonist for a second scene, centered around a particular content intended to help the second protagonist. While the director needs to understand group work, the group's gains will always be secondary and dependent on the protagonist's work.

Drama therapy was also developed by theater people. The following is an overview of its development in the United States; it is pared down to a few telling developments in order to introduce the reader to this relative newcomer in the world of therapy. Drama therapy has been developed in many other countries as well. The reader is encouraged to flesh out this brief overview with a wider exploration of the literature.

In the United States, a number of former actors and directors became psychotherapists and developed their theatrical skills to enhance their therapeutic regimen. David Johnson, Robert Landy, and Renee Emunah, as well as the author, all worked in the theater and found that its healing possibilities far outweighed the stress of a professional life exclusively devoted to it. Psychodrama had developed role theory: the hypothesis that the personality does not consist of a single, authentic self but rather of a whole cast of characters, some latent, some expressed. Drama therapy developed it further making use of Object Relations theory (Johnson) and humanistic psychology (Emunah), as well as the whole wide taxonomy of theatrical roles (Landy). Psychodrama used the various levels of the stage, lighting, and the improvisational skill of the actor to achieve its goals. Drama therapy added the group experience developed in drama class and in rehearsal, the heightened expression of performance, as well as many of the newer improvisational techniques.

While the psychodrama group concentrates its efforts on the protagonists's story, enriched with surplus reality and metaphor, the drama therapy group often begins in the fictitious realm with the goal of developing the entire group's spontaneity skills. In my view, drama therapy's most interesting theoretical contribution is the concept of distance—the degree of identification of the player with her role. Before drama therapy, actors thought in terms of styles of acting: the method actor approached her part directly, while the more classically trained actor might approach the part more exclusively through the role itself, a study of the role's (and play's) history, of movement and manners, and thus develop a greater sense of distance. The older actor thought of himself as portraying someone else—he may or may not have found similarities between himself and his character. The modern actor is always aware of the use she makes of parts of her own personality in order to play a role.

In the 1920's and 1930's when the Stanislawsky method began, acting became synonymous with the direct use of the actor's own experience. It was only when drama therapy came along that the possibilities of playing with the distance from a role was articulated. The use of fictitious roles, for example, allows a maximum of distance for those new to drama therapy, allowing them to interact with a sense of freedom from personal disclosure. Psychodrama may use theater games during the warm-up phase. Drama therapy may use theater games for several weeks until the whole group is warmed up to the possibility of more personal work. A group of adolescents, for example may have a wonderful time exploring fictional scenes of drug users, dealers, and the police, long before a particular member's drug use is brought up. Psychodrama uses the warm-up to discover the protagonist. Drama therapy uses the warm-ups to discover themes that the entire group can use as its members gradually become more self-disclosing. Whereas a warm-up in a geriatric group using psychodrama may lead to the selection of a protagonist who works on her fear of death, the same warm-up in a drama therapy group may lead to a group improvisation located in the sick ward of a retirement home.

A psychodrama is complete in itself. It has a beginning, middle and end. A drama therapy group may continue its development from week to week. This is perhaps best illustrated by the self-revelatory performance. In Renee Emunah's Drama Therapy Program, for example, students who study drama therapy technique develop five-to-ten minute performances designed to show an aspect of their own lives using theatrical metaphor, staging, props and other actors if they wish. Interestingly enough, the students, who can choose to do a self-revelatory performance as part of their Master's Thesis requirement, often extend this five-minute exercise to an hour's performance. The use of drama to express one's own life can yield a rich harvest of active introspection, growing insight, and the discharge of pent-up emotion—all of which lead to personal change and growth.

Drama therapy groups have also developed improvised plays on such subjects as substance abuse, imprisonment, teen-age gangs, and HIV infection and performed them for schools, parent-teachers' associations, clubs and other educational venues. These plays are often used to stimulate audience interaction. The play may be stopped during or after a significant scene, and the audience members invited to express their opinion about the content by stepping in, to change the scene, to ask the cast to play it differently, or to suggest a new scene.

One of the most interesting developments of therapeutic improvisational technique has been David Johnson's method of Developmental Transformations, in which there is a free-flowing change of content among group members and therapist(s) or between therapist and client. In this technique, any improvisation can be changed to a different content at any moment, the only rule being that the others have to agree. In other words, a married couple may be arguing about who takes out the garbage at one point, when the wife changes herself to a student and accuses her husband of being an unfair teacher. He then takes her offer and cooperates in the new scene, which, in turn, may shortly be transformed by him to one where he plays a young child asking her to join him in running away from school. There is, of course, much more to Johnson's method—but even a short example illustrates a new fluidity, akin to free association, which allows the unconscious to enter the realm of theatrical play.

Robert Landy has enriched the field of drama therapy with his concept of role distance and with a detailed investigation of theatrical roles. He describes individual work which may never leave the theatrical context, using a given role, such as Hamlet, by exploring its text and improvising and writing variations, to investigate personal difficulties without necessarily naming them.

Interestingly, the culmination of drama therapy can be a classic psychodrama. In Rene Emunah's stage-related drama therapy, she sees the development of the group in the following stages: 1) dramatic play, 2) scene work, 3) role play, 4) culminating enactment, and 5) dramatic ritual. Only stage three suggests the shift from the dramatic, fictitious play to role-playing actual events from the participants' lives. Stage four, the culminating enactment, shifts to the intense individual work of psychodrama.

Another innovation contributed by drama therapy is the use of ritual. Renee Emunah's stage five incorporates drama, poetry, musical instruments, and movement to bring the group's work—after a period of several months—to closure. Group members develop a ritual that helps make the transition from drama therapy skills ac-

quired in the group to using them in the outside world. David
Johnson's work with Viet Nam Veterans makes use of inpatients and
staff in a graduation ritual that incorporates individual grief, choral
responses, and dramatic readings in a ceremony that brings the
veterans the honor and dignity they deserve.

While both disciplines use props, drama therapy has used them
more extensively. The leader often equips the room with a variety
of objects: candles to use in rituals, photos of different historical
eras, props like small cars, bits of lace, toys, dolls, stuffed animals,
masks that can be used to evoke memories, stimulate enactments,
or set in a time line. Drama therapists have extended the use of
scarves not just for costumes, but to symbolize a bit of scenery such
as a wall, to represent a ghost, a particular aspect of the personality,
or even an atmosphere such as sunshine or dark night.

The similarities of the two discipline are great. Both need leaders
who are trained in group work and clinical skills. Both depend on
the use of theatrical techniques. Leaders need to understand the
tele, or group relationships, of their clients. Both leaders need to
be open to what the group members contribute so that the groups
can fulfill the functions the groups need, rather than those the
leader desires. The members of either group must be willing to use
the imagination, to play out themes in their own lives, rather than
following social convention and limiting themselves to talking about
these events. The magic of theater, when applied to therapy, is
capable of transforming the therapist, the clients, and the environment where the work is done.

Both psychodrama and drama therapy continue to develop and to
grow. Together, they enliven and enrich the field of psychotherapy.

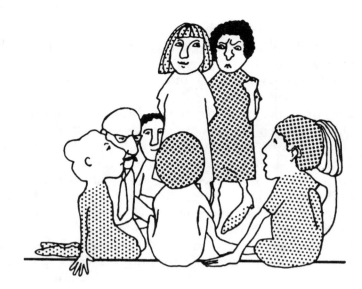

16

Closure

Moreno felt that one of the most important phases of a psychodrama is the sharing that takes place after the enactment. "They [the protagonist and auxiliaries] have given us much," he would say, "and they have the right to expect something from us. Remember that it is the function of group members to return the love which the protagonist has given" (in Fox p. 153). When the enactment has ended satisfactorily, all that is needed is the period of de-roling and sharing. When the protagonist and the audience share of feeling of incompleteness at the end of an enactment, the director must find a way to achieve closure. This chapter discusses some ways to achieve a feeling of completion in such a group.

In the days before psychodrama training had been formalized to the degree that it is today, practitioners often neglected the sharing phase and ended the enactment with applause. My own thoughts on this topic reflect my own encounters with the question of how to end psychodrama sessions. Today's training programs teach Moreno's methods in a thorough and systematic manner and obviate the need for such struggles. The following is presented for those who lack such training.

Life teaches us that it is much easier to set up a dramatic situation than to resolve it; the lesson holds for psychodrama as well. A volunteer from the audience is led through significant scenes in her childhood to a point where she has to make a confrontation—with a dead parent, a spouse, a boss, an employee, a friend—whom she wronged. The volunteer confronts the issue with drive and passion. As the scene climaxes, she dissolves into tears. Her auxiliary has nothing more to say in her role. The director lets the audience know that the psychodrama is over. The audience applauds and files out of the room. There is a sense of excitement; yet there is also a sense of unfinished business. Many leave wondering who will put Humpty-Dumpty back together again. Confronted by questions about the consequences of such a conclusion, a director may argue that the catharsis of the drama is healing enough. Talking about what happened would only dilute the experience. The clinician who observes this scene, may find herself thinking *I couldn't do that! He's just here for one session to demonstrate this technique. Then he leaves. I have to keep working with the people I see. I have to pick up the pieces. And he didn't show me anything about how to do that.*

The experience described above has been related to me many times during my work in teaching psychodrama to professionals. *What if I did get the courage to set up a psychodrama, only to find out I didn't know how to end it? Everyone knows there's a warm-up before the psychodrama begins. Is there some way to make the transition from the personal drama of the protagonist back to the group process? Is there a way to end with a feeling of resolution? How can I build trust in the protagonist and the rest of the group members?* These are legitimate questions for the group leader who may use psychodrama as only one among many other techniques.

One problem inherent in the psychodramatic process is that once dramatized, a situation may appear even more powerfully insoluble. The audience identifies with the protagonist, becomes emotionally rooted to her spot and, once the scene is played out, feels as helpless as she does. At the same time, the protagonist is making the transition from an emotionally involving, often intimate scene back to the group situation. She may feel vulnerable, confused, and in need of support from the group.

Resolution and closure are different processes. The resolution of a problem is a process that takes place on many different levels and over time. When a family conflict is portrayed, for example, partial resolution is accomplished just because the scene is enacted. The protagonist often finds relief in the dramatic expression of her problem. Airing the difficulty in front of empathic witnesses provides relief and may lend a new clarity. The emotional release that accompanies an enactment may enable the protagonist to see things in a different light. Another part of the resolution may come from an alternative solution suggested to her by a group member. But because the psychodrama is by its very nature an experiment, these resolutions can only be partial. They can point a direction; they can ease pain—but the true resolving must be done in real life.

Closure, on the other hand, is something the director can achieve. It refers to the feeling of completion after some work has been accomplished. The first part of closure requires the de-roling of the protagonist and the auxiliaries. Directors may ask those who contributed to the enactment to physically shake off the roles and/ or the emotions and then ask the auxiliaries to tell the protagonist what it was like to play the role, what was experienced both while playing the role, and in the split off part of the auxiliary that was observing the process. After shaking off the role, an auxiliary may say, for example, "I felt honored that you chose me to play your mom. When I was in the role, I could only see you as the problem in my life. I felt so out of control. As myself, I could really empathize. My mom was a lot like that."

Sharing with the other group members is the second part of the closure process. This process needs structure from the director. Two pitfalls come to mind. The first can be seen in the scene already described, which often leaves the protagonist without the comfort of sharing with her audience. At best, the protagonist is left strongly in touch with her emotions, and we can hope that this state will lead her to find a way of dealing with the problem she presented. At worst, the protagonist feels vulnerable and exploited. She doesn't know what the audience members intend by applauding. Do they find her dilemma entertaining? Do they like her despite her problems? Because of her problems? Do they feel sorry for her?

The second pitfall is created by our intolerance for the feeling of helplessness which can affect an audience after witnessing a poignant human dilemma. In their attempt to master this feeling of help-lessness, group members often adopt an artificially self-confident stance. The group starts intellectualizing. After witnessing a scene with a rejecting mother, audience members bombard the protagonist with questions: "When did you first feel this way? Did your mother treat the other children the same way? Did your mother ever praise you?" I refer to this maneuver as the group game of "Mr. District Attorney." The protagonist may answer despite the fact that she often finds herself becoming more confused. The group members may want to suggest alternative solutions: "Have you tried moving away from home? . . . Why don't you just tell your mother off and walk out? . . . I think you should stop blaming your mother, nobody's perfect. . . . Try just saying nothing when she talks like that, just let her talk." This is the group's version of the game "Psychiatrist," a game which leaves the protagonist feeling that everyone else in the group could handle her problem—only she apparently found it impossible. Both "Mr. District Attorney" and "Psychiatrist" create new problems for the protagonist.

Often the enactment will develop in a way that shows the director how the process of closure can proceed. Many enactments suggest, in the end, that several alternative solutions can be explored psycho-dramatically, giving the protagonist a chance to practice a new way of handling her problem with support from the group.

For example, a group member working on an intense conflict concerning her husband and another woman can finish by enacting resolutions which take place one year in the future: (1) if she takes a stand and her husband accepts it and stays; (2) if she takes a stand and the husband leaves (acting as if it is ten months since he left); and (3) if she takes no stand and keeps going along with the situation. Or, a young man with conflicts about leaving his mother may profit by setting up a scene during which his family discusses his sudden departure and another in which he talks to his own conscience about his feelings about having stayed another year. The director may want to explore alternative solutions by asking the protagonist to repeat a given scene using an alternative approach; i.e., if he has been passive and quiet in talking with his mother, he could now try an explicit, verbal approach. Often a feeling of completeness follows the exploration of alternatives. The individual is no longer viewed as a man trapped in an impossible dilemma: he has a number of alternatives to weigh and choose from; it is up to him to find a way that fits. Afterwards, group members can be encouraged to relate the part of the scene that touched them emotionally, and the group can leave, most of its business completed.

An incomplete enactment may not permit the investigation of alternative solution. Because time is short or because the protagonist is emotionally exhausted, the exploration of alternatives may not fit. At such times group members may be left with strong feelings of incompleteness. The protagonist and his fellow group members will need help to integrate the material evoked by the scene. In order to avoid the pitfalls of Mr. District Attorney and Psychiatrist, I structure the discussion in one of the following ways. I may use the collective double (described more fully in Chapter 4). Briefly, this technique involves the director saying something on the order of: "I see that there's still a lot of strong feeling here. While we were doing the scene I noticed sighs and some tears. How about putting yourself into the scene and speaking as one of the characters. Say what you might have said, or what you might want to say now, but first tell us who you are in the scene. For example, since this was Bob's scene, you might say, 'I'm Bob and I still feel angry at Mom.' Or, 'I'm Bob's mom and I just don't think Bob loves me any more.' "

The group tension lessens as different group members play out their feelings. The protagonist is supported by others speaking directly to his emotions. Group members have an opportunity to put their unresolved feelings into words.

The question "What touched you in what you just saw?" is also helpful. When I consult with groups accustomed to intellectual exchange—discussion groups, study groups, therapy groups—I usually make a point of delaying any discussion about what happened until after there has been an opportunity to respond to the protagonist. I say, "I know you may want to do some talking about the techniques I used or about some other aspects of the scene you just saw, but right now I don't want you to get away from your feelings. I know that most of you were very much involved in what was happening in the scene. Could you say what touched you?" I usually encourage group members to make short personal statements directly to the protagonist. If I find that someone wants to go further, I will usually say, "It sounds like you have something to work on in the same area Why don't you think about it, and if it still fits, we could work on

it next week." We want to avoid an intellectual response, such as
Mary saying, "I never knew John was the kind of person who felt so
deeply about his family." We don't want to give permission to gossip
about John in his presence. But when Mary says to John, "I was
touched by how much feeling you had for your family. I'd never
heard you talk that way before," John gets the direct support he needs
and the group tele is positively affected. My goal in the discussion
following psychodramatic work is to clear the decks, to leave with
as little unfinished business as possible.

Most of the time, the process described above leads to a feeling
of closure. Although no solutions have been reached, group members have had a chance to express their feelings and to explore briefly
the enactment's relevance to their own lives. The group member has
made the transition from feeling "this is John's crisis and it needs
an immediate solution," to "this feeling of crisis and frustration
occurs in my own life too. Here is an area where I have to do more
work. There are a lot of us with similar feelings in this group."

Occasionally, however, there is no time for group discussion, or
the discussion is not satisfactory. John, for example—especially if he
is a member of a low functioning group—may continue to look
confused and upset no matter what anyone says, leaving the other
group members frustrated and helpless. One or more group members may refuse to abide by the rules I set for the discussion—John
is attacked with criticism, suggestions, questions. Or a group member
may become upset and weep uncontrollably and/or abruptly leave
the room. When such problems arise, the director's first priority is
talk openly about her own feeling of incompleteness. The director
can state that, although the time of the group is almost over, the
work feels unfinished. She can let the group members know that
she doesn't expect to complete every enactment, that an incomplete
situation doesn't necessarily spell failure. The director may be able
to help make plans for an individual left with unresolved feelings.
Comments I make at such times may be, "We're going to have to
stop, and I know that there is a lot of work still to be done. Let's
see, John, you look like you're still kind of confused about what
happened. Is there someone you can talk with about that before we
meet next week?" (If John has a therapist, plans may be made to
talk further with him, if not I may suggest that he call another group
member or that he come in to see me for a short session mid-week.)

In a group at a day center or psychiatric ward, I may be able to suggest that a staff member present in the group be available for further contact. In a higher functioning group, I may say, "Sometimes, working like this leads us to an impasse and we're all left feeling various degrees of frustration. As much as possible, I'd like you to try to stay with that feeling of frustration. The more you get to know it, even if it is uncomfortable, the more you'll learn about your own impasse." After someone has left abruptly, I may say, "I know some of the feeling right now is for Barbara, because she got so upset and left the room. Does anyone want to go after her? Is anyone going to be seeing her? Or do you feel you can trust her to know what's right for her? I would like someone in the group to let her know that we hope she'll be back here with us next week. Who wants to do it? I can see some of you are still feeling how incomplete this session was. I'm still feeling some confusion about it also. Let's see what we do with these feelings as the week goes by and check in next time." When the enactment has further to go but there is no more time, I may say, "We have to stop, and I know there still is a lot more to say and explore. For now, we'll have to leave it the way it is, unfinished. This kind of session is not unusual in a psychodrama and often is very productive. I'll see you next week."

With these comments, the director gives the message that she continues to be in charge and that she is aware of the negative feelings and prepared to deal with them to some extent. Her goal is that the group members leave feeling a measure of support in a difficult situation.

High expectations often impede the director's effectiveness. *I should be able to cure every member of the group. I should run a group that goes smoothly, especially at the end. If it doesn't, I should keep working until everything is settled.* Only a gargantuan ego makes such demands—but the younger and the more inexperienced we are, the more we harbor perfectionistic demands. With more experience, the clinician will rid himself of his need to master every situation, to bring each conflict to resolution. Paradoxically, he will then experience more self-assurance. Once he can let go of the ideal situation, he will be freer to deal with the actual one.

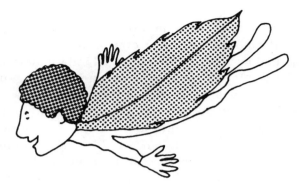

17

Psychodramatic Techniques in Use: Three Examples

The preceding pages have been devoted to the use of specific psycho-dramatic techniques. I want to close this book by relating three examples of my work in some detail. You will recognize the techniques; I will assume that they no longer need explanation. Here, I want to acquaint the reader with my own style and to convey, if possible, its underlying process revealing thought and feeling, and the intense absorption and excitement of a psychodrama group. This section is written in the hope that you will get a feeling for the work as a whole.

A PSYCHIATRIC WARD GROUP

The setting is the psychiatric ward of a large hospital in San Francisco. I go there once a week to conduct a psychodrama group. The clients remain at the hospital from two or three days to three or four weeks.

Some know me. Some don't. As we walk down the long corridors of the hospital to the group room, we sit in a circle where we are joined by other staff members. I tell the new ones my name and ask theirs. One of the clients puts a welcoming arm around me. After chatting a bit with the clients, we sit in a circle. The attending staff arrives; Judy, a rehabilitation counselor who has had some psychodrama training and attends our sessions regularly; Bob, a resident, verbal outgoing, and so eager to interact with the clients that I occasionally have to rein him in to keep his own problems from dominating the group; and Marie, a student nurse who blushes with shyness whenever she speaks. I look around the group. Nothing much is happening. People are looking straight ahead or down at the floor. *Here goes another meeting. Here goes nothing.*

I start to speak. "I'd like you to think of someone who knows you very well. An important person in your life, like a member of your family, someone you're living with, a close friend. I'm going to ask you to play the role of that person and describe yourself." *Such abstract words to describe such a simple, concrete task.* "Martha, you have an Aunt Jane. Be Aunt Jane telling us what a nuisance that Martha can be when she just won't do anything!" *We all know about Martha's Aunt Jane. This is a pretty safe start. Should I demonstrate? No, they can take it from here.*

Valerie, a young group member elegantly dressed in black, is willing to start. "I'm my friend Betty Ann. 'Valerie, you're so naive. You just don't know what you're talking about most of the time, and at your age, too!' " I ask her to stay in the role of Betty Ann and tell us more about Valerie. "Well, she's just so naive, she'll believe a promise from her boyfriend no matter how many times he's broken it. And she's stubborn! And shy. And very strong, too." I thank her. *We could start to work now, do a scene with Valerie and her boyfriend, but this is the warm-up and I want to hear from the others.*

We go around the circle because I sense that it will be easier than to wait for people to speak as they're ready. As we begin, each person gives a response. *No resistance to speak of. No newcomers in this group. And they like the work.*

Mary Jo is a young woman of Italian background in her twenties. She's been in and out of mental hospitals since she was a child, "I'm my sister Toni. 'Well, Mary Jo is all right but she gets so depressed so easily. I wish she'd just take her pills and get over her depression.' "

Turning to the group, "See that's all she thinks I have to do, just take my pills. 'Mary Jo is alone to much. She ought to get married again and forget about all that mental stuff.' "

Linda, a thirty-year-old black woman and obese, "I'm my step-mother. She's running down the stairs and then she opens the door and sees me. 'Oh, no, there's that girl again. She just bugs the life out of me, always hanging around her father. He doesn't want a girl that age hanging around that much. She just doesn't understand a thing!' "

A disgruntled-looking long-haired man in his late thirties: "Steve is selfish. I'm his wife and I can't get through to him. He's got a lot of problems and that's all he thinks about."

The resident (a rule in my groups is that everyone works, staff included). "I'm a friend of mine named Polly. 'Bob wants to work all the time. I just don't understand it. Why doesn't he come to Sausalito and enjoy life and sit around a little. Work, work, work.' "

We've gone most of the way around when a middle-aged woman in slacks, with untidy hair and a forbidding facial expression says: "I can't do it." *I should have known. Here's the resistance.* I repeat the task to her, suggest that maybe she could do it but doesn't want to, get her to talk about her husband a little, but she remains adamant: "I can't do it today." *At least we talked. She won't affect the rest of them as far as I can see. The paradox for the client: I'm sick, I'm helpless. How can they expect me to do something about my problems? How can they expect a helpless person to do anything?*

Jim, a middle-aged, obese, robust-looking man: "I'm my daughter Helen. She's twenty. 'Why can't it be like it used to be with my dad? When he worked, we all lived together and we went to the park and on picnics and we had a lot of fun. I want him to get a job so we can get an apartment and live together.' "

There are fourteen in the group, but Jim is the one I pick to start working. He has an urgency in his voice; he seems to want to say more. I know there are other clients in the room for whom the father-daughter issue is crucial. Earlier, the nurse told me that Mary Jo's father was dying of Hodgkin's disease, but she hadn't been able to talk about it at all. We heard Linda talking about her stepmother-father problem earlier.

Jim agrees that he'd like to continue the dialogue with Helen, his daughter. *I could let Mary Jo start—I have a feeling Jim would cast her, but I believe it's too soon for her. She might take the scene away from*

Jim and start to cry. Not yet. I want the scene to start out strongly and safely. Therefore, I ask Judy, the rehabilitation counselor, to take her role. I instruct them both to move their chairs into the middle of the circle. Judy (in the role of Helen) looks small, crestfallen.

Judy-Helen: When's it going to happen, Dad? You know how great things used to be for us. We did so much together. When are we going to be able to get an apartment?

Jim: When I get a job. You know I'm looking every day.

Helen: Are you really?

Jim: Yes, you know I want us to get together as much as you do. I'm confident that it'll all work out shortly.

I ask them to stop the scene for a moment. *I'm skeptical about what Jim is saying. He says he's taking so much responsibility. He's going to make it all work out right and here he is, in a hospital. He could be conning. I suspect he's furious at his daughter underneath.* "Could the two of you tune in to what you're feeling about each other and not saying? Turn to us and tell us some of your secret thoughts."

Jim: Well, I think she's right. It's time for me to get a job and . . . and work steady again and I want to do what's right for her.

Eva: (*He's not telling me how he feels. I ask him again.*) What are you feeling about all that?

Jim: Well it would be better if we lived together.

Eva: And how does that make you feel, what's it like for you to be talking with her?

Jim: It makes me feel awful. Like a failure.

(*I thank him and ask Helen to give us her secret thoughts.*)

Judy-Helen: I really want to live with him, but it's been so long. I'm getting tired of waiting. He hasn't had a full-time job in two years. Sometimes I think I shouldn't be waiting for Dad, that I should be out looking for a husband, to remarry. Maybe that's what I ought to do. I don't know.

I tell Judy to come back and sit in the circle and I go over to Jim. "I'd like you to think out loud about this for a minute, and I'd like to help you by talking with you as part of you, sort of another voice inside you." He agrees and I begin to double for him.

Double:	I wish my daughter would really talk like that, but she never says she wants to be on her own.
Jim:	Yeah, I wish she were more independent. She really shouldn't be living with me.
Double:	Would I ever tell her that?
Jim:	No. It would be hard. And I would like it if I could get a job and we could both live better.
Double:	Am I going to get a job?
Jim:	Oh, definitely. I'm really looking for one.
Double:	I'm conning now. I don't look that hard.
Jim:	No, I'm not conning. I don't have the money for transportation to look every day, but I'd say I look four times a week.
Double:	How long since I had a job?
Jim:	About ten months. (*He's approaching the truth slowly—I know it's been two years*)
Double:	Does it really look like it'll change?
Jim:	Well, not in my line as a draughtsman. I'd probably just get something temporary again, but I'd have to change my whole area of job capacity.
Double:	(*He's using impressive language. He sounds like a salesman*) I'm really conning now, always trying to reassure myself and my daughter.
	(*Jim sighs deeply and looks at me and smiles, shaking his head.*)
	(*Doubling, I imitate his gestures. We both laugh.*)

I ask Jim to talk to his daughter Helen one more time, cueing Judy to play the role as Jim describes it—dependent, hopeful that she'll be able to live with Jim. Stammering a little, he tells her that living together might not be so good after all. She's young. "Let's get our own lives straight. Just meet for dinners and stuff, that would be better."

Watching Jim, I feel he's still doing a good bit of conning. Saying what the therapist thinks is right. It looks as though it's what he wants to say for himself as well, but would he have the courage to say it in the real situation? I doubt it. Two more people stringing each other along on false promises. Anything rather than face one's failings. Anything.

The group members comment. I discourage questions and advice because I don't want to help the group members pretend that there are simple answers. I ask for feelings. What touched you? What was it like for you? Does Jim's situation strike a chord in you—a similar bind, a similar situation? Mary Jo looks at Jim. "You know, it's hard for kids when their parents suffer. I know when my folks are in trouble I'd do anything to stop it." Her voice is trembling a little, "your daughter probably thinks you can't take care of yourself since you split up with your wife. She wants to help you; be the wife you don't have." For the first time, Jim look genuinely moved. He nods.

I remember that Mary Jo's father is dying of Hodgkin's disease and that Mary Jo has said nothing about this during two hospitalizations within six months. Now I ask Mary Jo about herself as a daughter. The words burst out of her, "I think about it all the time. If one of them dies, I'm the one that has to take care of them. They're old and helpless. I couldn't leave them alone. My brother wouldn't do it. He never did give a damn. And my sister has her own family to take care of. I think and think about what it would be like growing old as a spinster, taking care of my dad, but I never get anywhere." *She is pretty and young; still, I could see her going through with it.* I ask her if she would like to do more work in this area by thinking out loud some more, with Judy as a double. I consider setting up a scene with her parents, but choose doubling because I want Mary Jo to confront herself, to get in touch with her own conflicting feelings. She agrees.

Mary Jo:	I don't even see them or talk to them that much but they're so good to me. My father sends me money. I don't even want him to but he still does and my mom really cares about how I'm doing.
Judy-Double:	I really feel I owe them something.
Mary Jo:	It's true. They've had such a hard life. My father's just this simple Italian and he worked like a dog all his life and then they bought this house just last year. After all the worries with us, one of the kids

died real early. This was finally going to be the re-
ward. They moved into this little beach house where
they are now and he's sick and she's getting weaker.
(*Her whole body is beginning to tremble.*) My dad can't
do anything for himself. He can't even boil an egg.

Judy-Double: I have to help. Somebody has to. I'll do it. I owe it
to them.

Mary Jo: I do. It was so hard for them all the time and I've
been going to hospitals with this trouble all my life.
I do owe him a lot. And when I picture one of them
helpless and see the lumps growing in my dad's
throat. . . . (*She's crying. It sounds as though she hasn't
cried in a long time; a high, screeching wail.*)

Linda gets up out of her chair and starts to walk across the room.
"I just can't stand to see anyone crying." Mary Jo gets up. "I'll stop.
I don't want to upset anybody." Marian, the nurse, quietly talks to
Linda and persuades her to stay, while I urge Mary Jo to continue.
She does.

Judy-Double: I can't bear to think of how helpless they are because
I feel so helpless myself so often.

Mary Jo: I think I'm the only one that knows what it's like.
But I really am. The others won't do anything and
they won't listen to me if I try to talk about it. I'm
the crazy one. I'm crazy. My sister even said it to
me.

Judy-Double: So I'm ready to give up my own life.

Mary Jo: (*sighs deeply*) I can't get out of it. I'm not getting
married again anyway. And I don't have any kids.
So I could do it.

Judy-Double: At least I love my parents. That's worth something.

Mary Jo: I do and they look so old and frail (*starts to cry again*).
They're in their seventies and they're going to be
dead. (*Cries.*)

*I'm sad for Mary Jo, but I'm glad that she's finally talking about her
parents' death. The particulars aren't important. It's enough that she dares
to open up to the frightening topic.*

Judy-Double:	(*waiting, letting Mary Jo's tears subside*) Why don't I count? There must be some way to be a good daughter and still live my own life.
Mary Jo:	It's true. I know that's right but I just don't know how to do it.
Judy-Double:	Maybe later. This is important now.

Mary Jo looks at me. "I want to stop now." I nod my head. *Mary Jo looks softer. She has stopped trembling. There is a quiet feeling in the room. Everyone in touch with the pain of watching someone else suffer, of helplessness. I ask the group members to relate what they're experiencing. Various people express empathy. I know they mean it. We were feeling with Mary Jo. And for ourselves.* Valerie says she was ready to do the same thing, just go back to Texas and take care of her folks.

Bob, the resident, reminds Mary Jo of her willingness to stop working in the middle of her scene because Linda was upset. "You count everyone else first."

I ask Mary Jo whether she has talked about her father with her own therapist. She replies that she's talked about it but it's been hard to get really close to what's bothering her, like today. Now she knows more clearly what she needs to talk about. She's going to ask her therapist to meet with her four times a week instead of three.

Valerie looks at Bob and Mary Jo. "You know, I've learned something today. I'm the same way. I always put everyone else first. I expect to be bothered and upset, but I don't think I ever have the right to bother anybody. Wow. I really learned something today."

I nod my head. *This has been a good beginning for Mary Jo.* "See you next week." The group is over.

A COUPLES GROUP

The group has been meeting once a week for three hours for the past seven months. The six couples know each other well. They work hard without the small talk and distraction that often characterizes group work. Many have made changes for the better. They've spurred each other on. My co-therapist and I use many experiential techniques in the group: role-playing, Gestalt dialogues, sensory awareness, and a television-feedback system run by a cameraman who has become a third therapist. The work often centers on individual growth. The initial period where the couple concentrates on the destructive marital games is often followed by individual work on the inner life, life goals and obstacles, and the family history.

Herbert tells us about his decision to take a leave of absence from a Ph.D. program in psychology. After promising a program of challenging experimentation with new techniques, the course turned out to be dull and conservative. Other group members express surprise. Herb is a lawyer who had impressed them with his plan to change careers. Now what? The session turns to a superficial question-and-answer game which I later label as a vocational counseling session. "How long is the leave of absence? . . . Do you think you'll really go back? . . . If you can't get your Ph.D. will you continue to practice law? . . . Aren't you afraid to just drop it? . . . You were so happy that you got into the program."

I'm not happy with what's going on. No feelings are coming out. Just a lot of talk. But they know that as well as l do. I try to tell myself that I don't have to make anything happen, just wait until something does. But it's hard on me when they don't work on deeper material. Herb comes through.

"I'm not getting anywhere. It's just like talking to my father: 'You need a career, Herb.' I used to think he was right but just don't anymore!" Herb's wife tells him that she thinks he's been closer to people since he's worked less. Herb agrees. "I sure talk a lot to my parents about it though. They think everything's going to be lost if I'm not a 'something.' They really panicked when I left the firm."

I feel relieved. Herb is getting into a real conflict within himself: a something versus a nothing. No wonder he's stuck. Maybe we can do some Gestalt work.

Eva:	All that small talk is beginning to make sense to me, Herb. And the fact that you took a leave of absence instead of quitting. It's as though you're suspended, not making a decision, not coming to terms with yourself in some way, and we've been suspended with you.
Herb:	It's that I really think I'm just going to totally drop out and then maybe I'll be happy. I don't know.
Eva:	How about a dialogue between Herb now and Herb the dropout. (*He is sitting on a pillow against the wall; I throw him another large pillow.*) Put the dropout Herb

	on the pillow there in front of you. Write a script between you and him.
Herb:	Wow . . . (*smiling and shaking his head*) you're really important to me. You're strong. I feel stuck here.
Eva:	Change pillows and get his reaction. (*He does.*)
Dropout:	You're scared, but you know better. You know you don't really need all that crap. Quit the games. Just be.
Herb:	Yeah, but you just tell me what not to do. So I quit the games? What then?
Dropout:	Wow . . . (*Herb turns to the group*). I'm really feeling scared. Really scared now.

I can feel his tension. I know he's on to something important. The group is so quiet you could hear a pin drop.

Eva:	How are you experiencing being scared?
Herb:	I can't seem to breathe very well. . . . And I feel shaky. I thought this was more than just a job crisis.

He really looks scared. I can feel it. So can other members of the group. Some are shifting in their seats. I feel excited. I don't know just where we're going but I know it's important. I hope I can handle it. The important thing is not to lead him. To take him wherever he's going. To follow him. Be in charge without being in control. It's hard when he looks so scared.

Eva:	Where in your body do you experience the shaking?
Herb:	It's not really shaking. Trembling. My upper body. My shoulders. My arms. (*Herb is tuning into himself now. It is obvious he no longer notices the other group members.*) I'm really scared.
Eva:	Shut your eyes and see if you can go into your fear. Give yourself a fantasy of what it's like. A landscape. An atmosphere.
Herb:	It's like floating. Like a leaf in the wind.
Eva:	(*Here it is: the metaphor I recognize as a messenger between conscious and unconscious, between body and soul. I was right earlier on, he really is suspended!*) Be the leaf. Tell us about your existence. Where you are. What you look like.

Herb:	I'm green and healthy and the wind is blowing me around. I'm floating all over the place and I'm being carried. (*Smiles.*) I like it. Just floating around. Nope. I'm afraid.
Eva:	What are you afraid of?
Herb:	I'm afraid I'm going to drop. I don't want to. I really don't want to drop. (*Smiling. He looks like he knows what he's saying—the metaphor of suspension is still being carried out.*)
Eva:	So drop. (*I'm smiling too, but I know I'm asking him to do something which isn't easy.*)
Herb:	I really don't want to. (*Still smiling.*) OK. Suddenly the wind stops carrying me. I drop to the ground. (*His face changes. He looks serious.*)
Eva:	What's it like there?
Herb:	I'm on the ground and I don't like it. I want to be back on the tree. I want to hold on. (*His voice is trembling.*)
Eva:	What's it like now? What do you look like?
Herb:	Brown. Shriveled up. (*He is trembling slightly.*) I don't want to go any further. (*Looking up at me.*)

This is it. What Fritz Perls called the death layer. Herb is really in it. I wonder if the others are feeling the same thing I am: he looks so shaken and so far away. How will he come out of this? No one makes any attempt to rescue Herb. My cotherapist looks at Herb.

Cotherapist:	You haven't finished yet. You still have further to go.
Herb:	Where?
Cotherapist:	Into the earth.

He's really putting it to Herb. I'm not sure I would have been so direct. But he's using Herb's metaphor and he's right.

Herb:	I know, but I'm not ready.

He can't deal directly with his own death. But we all know that he's looking at it more closely than he ever has.

Eva:	What are you feeling now?
Herb:	Cold. And very, very lonely.
Eva:	What happened to the trembling?
Herb:	It's gone. I feel quiet now. A stillness inside me. Very quiet and still.

I look around the group. Herb's words have a lot of meaning to each of us. Alone. Quiet. Still. They're hard to face, those words. I want to help Herb work through the metaphor of the leaf without invading his still, alone place. I still don't know how he'll come back to us.

Eva:	Talk to your stillness.
Herb:	I know you but I'm not ready for you.
Stillness:	I'm very large. I'm here. I'm waiting for you.
Herb:	I know, but I'm not ready. I still have a lot of things I want to do.

Herb is not looking at anyone. He is alone. I ask him whether he can come back to the group, to take a look at us. *He obliges, but I see that he isn't making any real contact yet. I have been noticing his wife every now and then during the work; she looked very involved. Now her eyes are full of feeling for Herb.* I ask Herb to take a look at Anne. *What follows is a rare moment of understanding. An intimate moment. He really sees her.* She looks at him, takes his hands, sees him withdraw slightly and lets him know in words that she has understood his struggle and felt some of it herself. *Realizing that I'm alone and that you're alone too: the words all marital games are designed to conceal. And the paradox. When the aloneness is faced deeply, togetherness is possible.* Herb and Anne are hugging. *There isn't a dry eye in the house. I feel a combination of relief and estrangement. The work is completed, but I've had to hold back my own feelings. That's as it should be. I'll deal with my own feelings about all this later.* I ask the other group members what the experience was like for them. Most of them express being deeply touched—by Herb showing us so honestly how alone we all are, by Herb's and Anne's togetherness, and the realization that the human condition is experienced so similarly by all of us. One group member says he lost track of what was going on early in the work and followed his own thoughts. *That's OK also. The group's comments allow me to get back to my own feelings again. I'm proud of Herb's courage and commitment. I'm satisfied with our work. Once begun, it developed so naturally. I feel deeply moved; there are tears in my eyes. There's a welcome sense of completion. The work has been good.*

ON SUPERVISION

As a therapist who has practiced both family therapy and psychodrama and as a supervisor of students, I am well aware of the effects that active, role-played supervision can have on a given institution. Psychodramatic enactments add a new dimension to the normal routine of staff meetings. Through role-playing, a past situation becomes part of the immediate present where group members can explore emotional reactions, call for empathy, and develop and practice alternative solutions. A novel aspect of on-site supervision in psychodrama is the changed role of the student intern, who, from being the new-comer or the least informed person in the system, is quickly transformed into the role of expert when it comes to role-playing. Supervising her will mean examining her changing role in the institutional system.

At a recent case conference attended by the creative arts interns, Mary, a student interning at Fairview, brought up her problems with George, a forty-year old moderately developmentally disabled man, who recently came out of a long depression because he has proposed marriage to his girlfriend, also developmentally delayed. With the encouragement of the student therapist, he was the first active participant in the group with a re-enactment of his proposal (his girlfriend is not a group member). The others, gathered in a semi-circle around the scene, had expressed enthusiastic praise mixed with a good deal of envy. During the discussion, Mary noticed to her surprise that George had his hands on another client's purse and was gently moving it closer to himself. She knew that George had been caught stealing before. At his girlfriend's mother's home, he had stolen some family photographs and a toy soldier in what could be interpreted as a touching attempt to join her family. He had been punished for the theft by being restricted to his residence at Fairview for two weeks. Now he seemed to be engaged in a further offense.

What to do? Mary, the intern, is in her twenties, unmarried, without the experience of raising children that might lend familiarity to such a situation. George is almost twenty years Mary's senior. When she observed his suspicious behavior, he had not stolen anything. *Not yet,* Mary thought. She was afraid of restricting George at this stage, afraid of being perceived as stern and forbidding and so she did nothing. A few minutes later, the purse was open and George's hand on the wallet inside. Now Mary had to act. "George, what are you doing?"

"Nothing," he answered, and looked down on his lap, having let go of the wallet as Mary spoke.

"You took my wallet," said Jane, the owner of the purse, a woman of George's age, easily upset and close to weeping.

George was silent. Mary, unsure of what to do next, told George that she would have to speak to other house staff about what happened, and, as time was up, proceeded with a closing circle during which the other group members appeared closed down and disturbed by what had happened. Mary herself felt inadequate and ashamed that she had let the situation get out of hand.

When Mary brought the incident to our case consultation, we had an opportunity not only to role-play different ways of handling George's behavior but also to begin to work on some of the differences that had caused dissonance in the system at Fairview. In the first part of our work, several enactments of the original scene enabled Mary to watch as others took her role and she played that of her client. What also emerged from the process was Mary's gradual discovery of new ways of handling the situation. She learned, through the others' example, that she could make a facial gesture that let George know she observed him. She could comment by clearing her throat to get George's attention without directly addressing what was going on. She could comment directly. In addition, the scenes helped her de-cathect the feeling of failure and 'stuckness' which she initially related to the group, as others commented on similar experiences in what I termed the conflict between wanting to play the positive role of helper and healer and a perceived negative role of disciplinarian.

With Mary taking the part of George and arranging some of the other participants as group members, one of the social workers demonstrated how she would handle the situation. She told us that when she first observed George's hand on Jane's purse, she would try to make eye-contact with George. In the enactment, George (played by our student intern, Mary) did not respond. What follows is the dialogue that ensued:

Social Worker:	George, what is happening?
Mary-George:	(*no response*)
Social Worker:	I just saw your hand on Jane's purse, George.
Mary-George:	I . . . nothing.
Social Worker:	(*in a kind voice*) Well, Jane's purse is pretty close to you and you could just get tempted to see what's in there, couldn't you?
Mary-George:	Well . . .
Social Worker:	And then it would be really easy just to touch it and maybe take it, huh?
Mary-George:	Well . . . yeah (*nods sheepish assent*)
Social Worker:	Listen, George, I don't want you to get into trouble and I know you don't want to get in trouble, so keep your hands to yourself, OK?
Mary-George:	(*nods again and moves away*).

Mary expressed a wish that she had been able to act earlier. She realized that she could take George's side in attempting to keep him out of trouble rather than having to oppose him by being the stern disciplinarian, the role she had been trying to avoid. In the discussion that followed, other clinical staff members also remarked on the social worker's gentleness and focused on how important it was to help George avert his unacceptable behavior in a supportive, non-punitive way.

The residential staff, however, was unified in expressing a different opinion which seemed to me to reflect a difference both in training and experience. While the clinical staff has graduate training in psychology and whatever specialty they represent, the residential staff is untrained. On the other hand, the clinical staff has less experience on the site, at most three or four years in comparison to the residential staff's average tenure of ten to twenty years. Added to this is the fact that a change has occurred in the general approach at Fairview over the last two years, where a more comprehensive clinical and creative arts approach has been added to a curriculum that was concentrated largely on basic maintenance and survival skills. Conflicts arise between the old and the new ways of working, between differences based on experience and training and reflected in the salary structure. While such activities as our case conference are intended to bring about better communication, there are times when the clinical staff and the residential staff polarize and take opposing views in relation to problem-solving and communication becomes adversarial. The atmosphere grew thick with tension during the first part of this discussion.

Members of the residential staff felt that Mary's problem with George should have been handled more directly. In fact, it was stated that the social worker's soft, gentle approach could have the effect of making George feel that what he was doing was alright. He needed to be told immediately that what he did was wrong. At this point, our student, Mary, was beginning to be worried about having brought up such an inflammatory subject and suggested we might want to go on to something else. The group, however, wanted to continue and my feeling, as I lead the group in the role-play that followed, was that we might be able to bring the opposing views closer together by maintaining our search for "collective wisdom" through role-play. Asked to demonstrate a more direct approach, the residential aide, an African-American woman who was also in her forties, showed us what she would have done.

Residential aide:	(*in a firm, slightly motherly tone that is not without warmth*) George, keep your hands to yourself.
Mary-George:	(*ignores her*)
Residential aide:	George, I told you. Keep your hands to yourself right now! You know that it's wrong to touch other people's stuff!
Mary-George:	(*puts his hands to his sides*)
Residential aide:	Now tell Jane you're sorry.
Mary-George:	I'm sorry.
Residential aide:	That's right, George, now I don't want to see that again, or you'll lose points, OK?
Mary-George:	OK.

The residential aide's voice was animated and strong as she set limits. Other staff members commented on how clear and direct her communication had been, and how much George could profit from hearing such a strong message. Clearly, George did not want to lose points which could be used to limit his freedom to move off-campus. The conflict was now clearly delineated. This was just the kind of language the clinical staff resisted. The tension in the room remained high. One of the clinicians commented, "It's great when you can set limits but if feels like being a little Hitler, you know?" and one of the residential aides answered, "We never do that. We don't act that way. We just set clear boundaries and teach them values."

My aim, in the discussion that followed, was to keep the group focused on the differing experiences of the aide and social worker facing the same situation—the consequences of having different roles in the system—particularly in the way they experienced their own responsibility and the need to control their clients. Group members talked about the almost parental responsibility the aides seemed to feel: since it was up to them to keep the dormitory residents to an orderly schedule of daily activities, they naturally became more frustrated with uncooperative clients. Clinical staff, on the other hand, saw their responsibilities as akin to more peripheral members of a family like a grandmother or aunt, who on visiting, could pay attention to a troubled family member and, through empathy and patience, bring about a better adjustment. Our student, Mary, became more and more thoughtful. She related that she had often felt privileged because she could come and go, whereas the residential staff had no recourse but to stay and keep dealing the conflict. Some of the residential staff members responded by accounts of the mounting stress of working full-time.

Our example illustrates that while there is the possibility of dealing with areas of greater conflict than in our usual settings, on-site supervision also provides us with rich opportunities to help our students understand their role in a complex professional system.

Epilogue

When I was developing the techniques in this book, the climate of psychotherapy was dominated by a psychoanalytic point of view. Therapy was commonly regarded as a process occurring between two people: a doctor and a client talking about the client's life. Only a few clinicians, clearly outside the mainstream, practiced anything different, such as group therapy and psychodrama.

In the late 1950s and early 1960s came the challengers, the change makers. From psychiatry, social work, sociology, psychology—disciplines that had been infused with knowledge from psychoanalysis and had much of their own to contribute—came individuals who explored new ways of doing psychotherapy. Times and symptoms were changing. More and more people were interested in psychotherapy. Instead of seeking help for symptoms such as hysterical paralysis, they often sought more elusive qualities such as "more effective functioning," "better communication," or simply "growth." The psychotherapy group came into prominent use. The one-to-one, exclusively verbal approach to psychotherapy began to recede from the dominant position it held for so many years.

Fritz Perls, Virginia Satir, Don Jackson, Jay Haley, and Stanley Keleman, and many other pioneers developed innovative techniques that highlighted immediate experiencing. Conjoint interviews of couples and families, anathema in conservative psychiatry, were explored by John Bell, Virginia Satir, and a few others. Earlier, Moreno in New York had developed psychodrama as a therapeutic tool and now his influence grew, as other therapists, I among them, developed their own methods. There seemed to be a wave of change washing over what had become an arid landscape. The revival of psychodrama was part of that wave.

As a consequence of the focus on experience, the scope of therapy broadened. Other disciplines helpful in expanding awareness and consciousness came into use as adjuncts to psychotherapy. Drama, dance, art, yoga, zen practice, mime, aikido, massage, video-feedback, and many more became a part of the therapeutic tool chest. The wave took on larger proportions. On it rode many therapists—now called group facilitators, leaders, or counselors—whose training in the specific new discipline was usually excellent but whose clinical skills were often limited to little more than enthusiasm and good will. I viewed their arrival with mixed feelings. They were young and enthusiastic, and brought new skills that enlivened and challenged the old regime. But could they do the job? Did they have any idea of the complexities of human relationships?

The early challengers (myself included) had respected the establishment they were challenging. They were well-trained, conscientious, frequently highly credentialed clinicians. What they did not foresee was that expanding therapeutic techniques and making them widely available could have a detrimental result: namely, that the highly valued discipline and knowledge of clinical skills which they possessed could no longer be taken for granted in other therapists.

What do I mean by clinical skills? I am referring to the skills that let us assess what is wrong and find a way to help it become less so. Clinical skills are the ground of our work. They include sensitivity to the moment, as well as a long-range understanding of what is normal and what is possible, and the ability to communicate effectively at the right time. The skilled clinician knows her own potential and can turn away the client whom she feels ill-equipped to treat. These skills cannot be developed quickly. They require years of devoted, intensive study of human beings—including the clinician herself—their patterns of growth, their inner processes, and their interrelationships— in a training program with the guidance and supervision of experienced clinicians.

When I began to write this book, I wanted primarily to encourage those clinicians—members of the old school—who were eager to try some of the newer techniques but too shy to do so. They knew a great deal, were often already successful in their practice when they came to me as students, and felt that experiential techniques would help them work in a more powerful, richer way. I wanted (and still want) to teach them that it is all right to role-play, to move chairs and desks, to explore in an active, spontaneous manner.

Recent change in psychotherapy has oriented me to another goal. I want to help the talented newcomers develop their clinical skills. Many of these new students have no fear of active techniques. Typical is the student who, during his first interview with a family, has them reverse roles, divide up into teams, each commenting on the other's behavior, and do breathing and relaxation exercises. His cup may run over with techniques, yet he experiences difficulties. Without academic discipline behind him, and lacking years of first-hand experience, he seems unable to understand what is happening in the contexts he so actively creates. He feels like a recreational counselor: he can set up activities and enliven the interview, but he lacks the skills with which he could help the family integrate these activities. He experiences neither the continuity of his hour nor closure at the end of it.

It is my hope that this book offers some help in developing clinical skills. The discussion of such concepts as doubling, closure, and resistances is intended to help a student integrate his techniques clinically, so that the experiences he arranges for his clients can do what they are supposed to do—lead to individual growth. In the last ten years, psychodrama has become a more and more familiar technique. It lends a richer, more exciting, and immediate experience to many of the issues facing the client, the therapist, and any others involved in his treatment. My hope is that this book will continue to further its use.

EVA LEVETON
June 1976

Since I wrote those words, I learned that the field of psychotherapy undergoes cyclical changes. A period characterized by the use of fantasy and imagination is followed by one in which students anxiously learn the "right" protocol, fearing the dangers of eclecticism.

Therapy, after all, reflects the values of the society in which it is conducted. As long as psychotherapy is considered an art as well as a science, there will be those who are interested in pursuing the paths of healing through active dramatic techniques. This book is written for their use.

EVA LEVETON
Spring 1991

The cycles of time turn and turn. At this writing, the field of mental health is once more dominated by the medical model with its emphasis on diagnosis and medication. But whereas in earlier times, the medically trained psychiatrist was the most powerful among therapists, this cycle has reduced his scope by making him subservient to health plans which limit his time and often reduce his work to diagnosis and prescription of psychotropic medicines. Reduced funding of state and federal mental institutions has all but replaced individual with group therapy. One interesting consequence of this process is that students graduating from programs that train group therapy skills are hired by public institutions because their work is cost-effective. Graduates of schools that teach psychodrama and drama therapy at the Master's level find themselves with the heavy responsibility of running groups in psychiatric hospitals, senior centers, schools, substance abuse clinics, and adolescent facilities.

Interestingly, in an overall conservative mental health setting, psychodrama has become one of the treatments of choice. It has become general knowledge that clients can regain spontaneity, develop their empathic attunement, and express their problems without risking confrontation with the actual cast of characters that troubles their lives. Problems can be shared and new skills practiced. Because of the shortage of staff, the group therapist often finds herself in charge of follow-up as well. Psychodramatic skills have been extended to use with individual clients.

Today's clinician is equipped with many skills that enhance talk therapy and fill the therapeutic hour with art, poetry, movement and drama. As my own development has drawn from drama therapy, I will include some of its literature in the revised bibliography. No longer timid, today's clinician can choose her techniques from a wide range of possibilities. My hope is that this volume will enhance her skills.

EVA LEVETON
March, 2001

Glossary

Many of the terms that follow are already familiar to the reader. I have not tried to define them in the conventional sense. A dictionary can be consulted for that purpose. Instead, I've tried to provide the reader with definitions and short explanations of words used in a peculiar way by psychodramatists, drama therapists, and theater folk. I've also tried to give the reader a very quick introduction to some of the individuals whose original work enhanced the progress of my eclecticism.

Acting. A discipline that trains the actor to take part in theater or film work. Acting is often confused with role playing, which is, in fact, only a small part of the discipline comprising improvisation, mime, voice production, body movement, character building, analysis of text, and many other techniques.

Auxiliary. Originally Moreno's "auxiliary ego" the term refers to the individuals who help the protagonist by taking parts in his drama.

Berne, Eric. Author of *Transactional Analysis in Psychotherapy and Games People Play*; founder of transactional analysis, a system of individual and group dynamics using group therapy.

Bridge. Used to describe the connection the leader makes between the various scenes in a psychodrama and the commentary that precedes and follows them.

Catharsis. The discharge of intense emotion through its expression in a psychodrama, as, for example, the expression of unexpressed grief or anger in a particular scene.

Childhood recall. Sometimes referred to as age regression, the vivid and detailed recall of childhood experiences not readily available to the individual.

Client. A person under sufficient stress to pay for the services of another to help reduce it.

Conflicts. The collisions of opposing forces that are the heart of psychodrama. Whether the struggle is inter- or intrapersonal, both sides of the conflict are enacted on the psychodramatic stage.

Control. Here used in the sense of an individual's ability to remain in charge of his emotions. The leader must be aware that unpredicted outbursts of tears or anger in an enactment may challenge a protagonist's or auxiliary's sense control.

Critical distance. The physical distance vis-a-vis others comfortable for the role-player.

Director. The person in charge of a specific psychodrama. (There may be several directors in a group where each scene has a different director.)

Distancing. Here used to mean (1) putting the other person off, at a psychological distance, or (2) viewing the material from a greater distance, as when the protagonist chooses to direct all or part of scene rather than take part in it, or (3) locating the other person in the physical distance that fits the perceived psychological relationship.

Double. An auxiliary who represents another part of the protagonist.

Enactment. The staging of a protagonist's scene.

Erickson, Milton, M.D. Hypnotist known for the development of clinical hypnosis using metaphor and story to help clients work on their problems while in a state of relaxation.

Encounter.   A psychotherapeutic approach centering on a dialogue between peers where each is expected to comment frankly and honestly on the other's behavior.

Drama therapy.   A discipline developed in the '80s using drama and theater-based techniques to further emotional growth and individual change. It differs from psychodrama in its more direct connection with theater and performance and its focus on the whole group rather than the protagonist.

Emunah, Renee.   Innovator of Drama Therapy. Author of *Acting for Real, Drama Therapy Process, Technique, and Performance.*

Esalen.   A spa with hot springs in Big Sur, California, used as a center for learning. Both Fritz Perls and Virginia Satir were long-term resident teachers there.

Experiential.   Here used to describe a therapeutic technique that actively provides the individual with a new life experience, as contrasted to the more analytic "talking" therapies.

Fantasy.   All role-playing requires fantasy, but here we refer to material outside the real life situation of the role player. A fantasy role is imagined in the sense that it takes place in another country, another life zone, or dreams; a person can change into an animal, a rock, a much richer or poorer individual, etc. Another term used for this category is surplus reality.

Gestalt.   A psychiatric theory and technique developed by Fritz Perls. *Gestalt,* the German word for figure, refers to the individual's need to complete his psychologically unfinished business, lest he spend his life repeating the same patterns, just as the hungry person spends his time with recurrent fantasies of food until his hunger is satisfied.

Haley, Jay.   Member of the original Mental Research Institute group that developed systems and communications theory and the concept of the double bind. Author of many books, including *Uncommon Therapy and Problem-Solving Therapy.*

High-functioning group. Term used to refer to a group that can function without being affected by major psychological or physical handicaps.

Humor. Here used to highlight the use of irony and humorous contrast in a psychodrama to help an individual see problems from a lighter perspective.

Impasse. A stuck place reached when an enactment begins to lose energy and become repetitive because its protagonist has reached a major internal obstacle.

Intellectualization. A psychological defense mechanism in which a threat is deprived of its emotional content through intellectual analysis.

Johnson, David. Pioneer of Drama Therapy. Author of many articles describing his developmental theory and innovative improvisational technique in drama therapy.

Jackson, Don. Member of the original Mental Research Institute (MRI), Palo Alto, California (see Jay Haley). Editor of *Human Communication, Volumes I and II*, a compendium of this group's work.

Keleman, Stan. Teacher of Bio-Energetics (a system combining body awareness and psychological dynamics), therapist, and author of *Living Your Dying*.

Korn, Richard. Practicing psychodramatist best known for his work with prison inmates and prison personnel; trained by J. L. Moreno.

Lewin, Kurt. Sociologist. Founder of Field Theory, a system of social psychology that stresses the necessity of considering context in the analysis of any situation.

Low-functioning group. A group whose members are severely handicapped psychiatrically, physically, or mentally. Because their handicaps will make it difficult to focus attention, to maintain control, to express themselves freely or easily, the director must provide more structure and more concrete directions than in high-functioning groups.

Magic shop.   Psychodramatic technique that uses the device of a shop dealing in human qualities to examine them.

Mirror.   Psychodramatic technique in which an auxiliary mimics the protagonist to demonstrate an aspect of behavior of which she is unaware.

Model.   To demonstrate how to play a role, comment, or behave spontaneously; an important aspect of psychodramatic leadership.

Moreno, J. L.   Founder of psychodrama as a system of psychiatric dynamics and a technique of teaching and psychotherapy. Author of *Psychodrama,* Vol. I and, together with Zerka Moreno, Vol. II and Vol. III, and coeditor with A. Friedemann, and R. Battegar of *The International Handbook of Group Therapy.* The Morenos are the originators of psychodrama and have published widely in addition to these seminal volumes.

Moreno, Zerka.   Psychodramatist, author, and coauthor with J. L. Moreno of *Psychodrama,* Vols. II and III, coeditor with J. L. Moreno, A. Friedemann, and R. Battegar of *The International Handbook of Group Therapy,* and with Dag Blomkvist, *Surplus Reality and the Art of Healing.*

Perls, Fritz.   Founder of Gestalt Therapy. Author of *Ego, Hunger and Aggression; Gestalt Therapy* (co-authors: Ralph Hefferline and Paul Goodman).

Process.   The "how" of doing something, here used to explore the workings of the director as well as the group interaction.

Protagonist.   The main character in a psychodrama.

Psychodrama.   Term originated by Moreno, which we use in a more general sense to designate role-playing in the service of personal growth.

Resistance.   In relation to psychodrama, the psychological defenses designed to protect the individual from the dangers of change by cooperating without commitment, refusing to cooperate, or otherwise sabotaging the goals of the director and the group.

Resolution.   The psychodrama achieves resolution when there is a lessening of tension and sense of completion that may be accompanied by a different point of view, a new solution, or insight.

Risk.   Used when a person takes a leap into the psychological unknown.

Ritual.   An activity that marks an important event or transition in human development, often conducted by a specialist such as a priest or a shaman. Psychodrama often takes on a ritual quality.

Role-playing.   Taking part in a psychodrama. It is important not to confuse role playing with acting. Role playing refers to spontaneous improvisation depending solely on the participant's ability to fit himself into the role and his reactions to the others. Acting, on the other hand, begins with role-playing but involves a complex discipline requiring the individual to be able to learn scripts, play in a way suitable for stage or film, and repeat performances in exact detail.

Role reversal.   When two role playing individuals take each other's roles. (In a father-son dialogue, for example, the father plays the son's part while the son plays the father.) For an excellent discussion of role reversal, see Adam Blatner, *Acting-In: Practical Applications of Psychodramatic Methods* (New York: Springer Publishing, 1988).

Satir, Virginia.   Author of *Conjoint Family Therapy* and *People Making.* A leader in the development of family therapy and the evolution of experiential techniques.

Sacred space.   A place where the ordinary world can be transcended. The psychodramatic stage often becomes a sacred space.

Scene.   A part of a psychodrama with a beginning and an end. Directors often find it useful to divide a psychodrama into various scenes, each with a specific purpose.

Sculpture. An experiential technique requiring an individual to shape another person (or persons) into the posture he feels appropriately describes an emotional relationship.

Sensory awareness. A therapeutic technique designed to provide the individual with greater information about his body and his five senses.

Sociodrama. Moreno's term for drama based on social issues facing the whole group, for example, racial conflicts in a group with both Caucasian and Black members.

Sociogram. A psychodramatic technique requiring the individual to make a living picture of a group of persons important to him by placing them at the physical distance appropriate for their psychological relationship.

Soliloqui. The protagonist speaks his thoughts directly to the audience.

Stage. Here used to designate any area where a psychodrama takes place.

Strategy. A plan developed by a psychodrama leader or director for a specific purpose in a particular psychodrama.

Style. The manner of doing one's work; that which is personal and idiosyncratic in the psychodrama director's performance.

Surplus reality. The world that takes place on the psychodramatic stage where anything can take place—time travel, fantasy, enacted metaphor—and still be seen in the present and in real dimensions.

Tele. Term coined by Moreno to denote the dynamic that determines the way in which individuals are connected in a group in terms of their attraction and repulsion. It accounts for preferences between group members, the mood of the group and the intuitive leaps often made in role assignments and role-playing.

Warm-up. The initial activity in a psychodrama group designed to encourage maximum participation and spontaneity as well as introduce material for further work.

between group members, the mood of the group and the intuitive leaps often made in role assignments and role-playing.

Warm-up.   The initial activity in a psychodrama group designed to encourage maximum participation and spontaneity as well as introduce material for further work.

Bibliography

Psychodrama

Blatner, A. (1996). *Acting-in: Practical applications of psychodramatic methods.* New York: Springer Publishing.

Blatner, A., & Blatner, A. (2000). *Foundations of psychodrama, history, theory, and practice.* New York: Springer Publishing.

Brazier, D. (1997). *Zen therapy, transcending the sorrows of the human mind.* New York: John Wiley and Sons.

Fox, J. (Ed.). (1987). *The essential Moreno: Writings on psychodrama, group method, and spontaneity.* New York: Springer Publishing.

Fox, J. (1986). *Acts of service: Spontaneity, commitment, tradition in the nonscripted theatre.* New Paltz, New York: Tusitala Publishing.

Holmes, P., & Karp, M. (Eds.), with drawings by Ken Sprague. (1991). *Psychodrama, inspiration and technique.* London: Routledge.

Journal of Group Psychotherapy, Psychodrama and Sociometry. Washington, DC: Heldref Publications.

Leveton, E. (1991). The use of doubling to counter resistance in family and individual treatment. In *The arts in psychotherapy, Vol. 18* (pp. 241–249). Pergamon Press.

Leveton, E. (1996). Is it therapy or what? Boundary issues between teacher and students of psychodrama and drama therapy in the context of single session therapy. In A. Gersie, *Dramatic approaches to brief therapy* (pp. 146–160). London: Jessica Kingsley.

Marineau, R. F. (1989). *Jactob Levy Moreno 1889–1974.* London: Tavistock/Routledge.

Moreno, J. L. (1977). *Psychodrama* (Vol. 1) (Rev. ed.). Beacon, New York: Beacon House.

Moreno, J. L. (1973). *The theatre of spontaneity.* Beacon, New York: Beacon House.

Moreno, J. L. (1975). *Psychodrama: Action therapy and principles of practice* (Vol. 3). Beacon, New York: Beacon House.

Moreno, J. L., & Moreno, Z. (1975). *Psychodrama* (Vol. 2). Beacon, New York: Beacon House.

Moreno, Z. T., Blomquist, L. D., & Rützel, T. (2000). *Psychodrama, surplus reality and the art of healing.* London: Routledge.

Sternberg, P., & Garcia, A. (1989). *Sociodrama, who's in your shoes?* New York: Praeger.

Williams, A. (1989). *The Passionate Technique; strategic psychodrama with individuals, families, and groups.* London: Tavistock/Routledge.

Yablonsky, L. (1975). *Psychodrama: Resolving emotional problems through role-playing.* New York: Basic Books.

Drama and Improvisation

Nachmanovitch, S. (1990). *Free play; improvisation in life and art.* New York: Jeremy P. Tarcher/Putnam, a member of Penguin Putnam Inc.

Spolin, V. (1963). *Improvisations for the theater.* Evanston, IL: Northwestern University Press.

Stanislavski, C. (1961). *Creating a role.* New York: Theatre Arts Books.

Wirth, J. (1995). *Interactive acting; acting, improvisation, and interacting for audience participatory theater.* Fall Creek, OR: Fall Creek Press.

Zaporah, R. (1995). *Action theater; the improvisation of presence.* Berkeley, CA: North Atlantic Books.

Drama Therapy

Boal, A. (1995). *The rainbow of desire: The boal method of theatre and therapy* (Adrian Jackson, tran.). New York: Urizen Books.

Cattanach, A. (1997). *Children's stories in play therapy.* London: Jessica Kingsley.

Dramatherapy, the journal of British Association of Drama Therapists. Manchester, England.

Emunah, R. (1994). *Acting for real; drama therapy, process, technique and performance.* New York: Bruner/Mazel.

Emunah, R. (1989). The use of dramatic enactment in the training of drama therapists. *The Arts in Psychotherapy*, Vol. 16 (pp. 29–36).

Gersie, A. (Ed.). (1996) *Dramatic approaches to brief therapy* (pp. 146–160). London: Jessica Kingsley.

Gersie, A., & King, N. (1990). *Storymaking in therapy and education.* London: Jessica Kingsley.

Jennings, S. (1990). *Dramatherapy with families, groups, and individuals: Waiting in the wings.* London: Jessica Kingsley.

Jennings, S. (1993). *Theatre, ritual and transformation.* London: Routledge.

Johnson, D. (1992). Drama therapy in role. In S. Jennings (Ed.), *Drama therapy, theory and practice* (Vol. II). London: Routledge.

Landy, R. (1993). *Persona and Performance; the meaning of role in theater, therapy and everyday life.* New York: The Guilford Press.

Leveton, E. (1996). Is it therapy or what? Boundary issues between teachers and students of psychodrama and drama therapy in the context of single session therapy. In A. Gersie (Ed.), *Dramatic approaches to brief therapy.* London: Jessica Kingsley.

The arts in psychotherapy. Pergamon Press, Elsevier Science, Inc., New York, NY.

Gestalt Therapy

Perls, F. (1973). *The Gestalt approach: Eyewitness to therapy.* Palo Alto, CA: Science and Behavior Books.

Hypnosis

Bandler, R., & Grinder, J. (1975). The structure of magic. Palo Alto, CA: Science and Behavior Books.

Haley, J. (1985). *Conversations with Milton H. Erickson, M.D.* (Vols. 1–3). New York: Triangle Press.

Haley, J. (1973). *Uncommon therapy: The techniques of Milton H. Erickson, M.D.* New York: Norton.

Mime

Rolfe, B. (1977). *Behind the mask.* Oakland, CA: Persona Products.

General

Berne, Eric (1996) *Games People Play,* New York: Penguin

Fixel, J. (1972). Personal Communication.

Jackson, Don (1968) Therapy, communication, and change, Palo Alto, California: Science & Behavior Books.

Keleman, Stanley (1985) *Emotional Anatomy.* Berkeley, California: Center Press.

Leveton, E. (1985). *Adolescent crisis: Approaches in family therapy.* New York: Springer Publishing.

Nisker, W. (1990). *Crazy wisdom.* Berkeley, CA: Ten Speed Press.

Satir, V. (1964). *Conjoint family therapy.* Palo Alto, CA: Science & Behavior Books.

Winnicott, D. W. (1990). *Playing and reality.* New York: Basic Books.

Winnicott, D. W. (1986). *Home is where we start from: Essays by a psychoanalyst.* New York: W. W. Norton.

Yalom, I. D. (1990). *The theory and practice of group therapy* (2nd ed.). New York: Basic Books, Inc.

Index

S